# 150 TIPS AND TRICKS for New Moms

From Those Frantic First Days to Baby's First Birthday—
Everything You Need to Know to Enjoy Your New Addition

Robin Elise Weiss, Certified Childbirth Educator

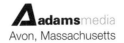

Avon, Massachusetts

Copyright © 2009 by F+W Media, Inc.
All rights reserved.
This book, or parts thereof, may not be reproduced in any
form without permission from the publisher; exceptions are
made for brief excerpts used in published reviews.

Published by
Adams Media, a division of F+W Media, Inc.
57 Littlefield Street, Avon, MA 02322. U.S.A.
*www.adamsmedia.com*

Contains material adapted and abridged from *The Everything® Mother's First
Year Book*, by Robin Elise Weiss, © 2005 by F+W Media, Inc.,
ISBN 10: 1-59337-425-9; ISBN 13: 978-1-59337-425-9.

ISBN 10: 1-60550-348-7
ISBN 13: 978-1-60550-348-6
Printed in the United States of America.

J I H G F E D C B A

**Library of Congress Cataloging-in-Publication Data**
is available from the publisher.

This publication is designed to provide accurate and authoritative information
with regard to the subject matter covered. It is sold with the understanding that
the publisher is not engaged in rendering legal, accounting, or other professional
advice. If legal advice or other expert assistance is required, the services of a
competent professional person should be sought.
 —From a *Declaration of Principles* jointly adopted by a Committee of the
American Bar Association and a Committee of Publishers and Associations

Many of the designations used by manufacturers and sellers to distinguish their
product are claimed as trademarks. Where those designations appear in this
book and Adams Media was aware of a trademark claim, the designations have
been printed with initial capital letters.

*This book is available at quantity discounts for bulk purchases.
For information, please call 1-800-289-0963.*

# Contents

Introduction • iv

Part One • 1
Pre-Baby Preparation

Part Two • 25
The Birth and Your First Weeks as a Mom

Part Three • 43
Baby Care Basics

Part Four • 61
Nutrition for the Family

Part Five • 79
Physical and Mental Development

Part Six • 101
Post-Baby Body and Fitness

Part Seven • 119
Sex after Baby

Part Eight •141
Working and Child Care

Part Nine • 161
Stay-at-Home Parenthood

Part Ten • 181
Ready for More?

Index • 199

# Introduction
## Becoming a Mom

The fact that you've picked up this book means that you are getting ready for one of the most exciting, challenging, and life-changing experiences a person can have: You're going to be a mom! You may be feeling anxious, worried, elated, or a combination of all three. Once your baby is born several more emotions (many of them hormone related) will work their way into the mix as well. One thing's for sure: Pregnancy and birth are a wild ride!

The good news is that feelings of anxiety and worry are completely normal as you prepare for parenthood. Rest assured that all the basic, practical information you need for when your baby comes is in this book. You'll find tips for choosing diapers and bottles, guidelines for nutrition and feeding, tricks for handling sleep issues, and myriad other helpful hints. One thing that you can't get from this or any book, however, is a recipe for your parenting style and goals. This is very personal to you and your partner as parents, and it's something you should seriously consider before your baby arrives.

As soon as your belly starts to blossom, words of advice will probably start flowing in from all directions. During pregnancy, excess advice may be easy to shrug off, as your baby has not yet arrived. But once the baby is born, you may be a little more likely to worry. Just remember to listen only to advice that seems to be practical. Think about how it might apply to your life. Does it make sense? How would you feel if you applied it? Does it go against any of your major beliefs about parenting?

If an idea seems to meet all your requirements, consider trying it out. Remember, you can always scrap the idea if it doesn't work for you.

Despite what anyone tells you, your parenting style must be developed over time—by you. However, you can still pick up tricks from existing parenting styles, including those that seem like fads. You can also take advice from friends and family—but with a grain of salt; a few of their methods might work for you, but others might not. Simply keep an open mind and consider your baby's unique characteristics when making these decisions.

Above all, remember that becoming a parent is a journey. You won't have all the answers the first week, the first month, or even the first year. As your family grows and evolves you'll continuously learn more about yourself, your partner, and your child. As long as you work together as a team and keep your child's best interests at heart, you can't go wrong. Congratulations, good luck, and enjoy this magical experience!

**1.** Decide Who Will be at the Birth • 2–3
**2.** Consider Important Delivery Details • 4
**3.** Take Childbirth Classes • 5
**4.** Pack for the Hospital • 6
**5.** Decide When to Leave Work • 7
**6.** Learn about Maternity Leave • 8–9
**7.** Budget for Baby • 10–11
**8.** Get Help and Stock Up • 12–13
**9.** Choose a Pediatrician • 14
**10.** Get a Car Seat • 15–16
**11.** Cribs, Bassinets, Cradles, and Co-sleepers • 17
**12.** Invest in a Stroller • 18–19
**13.** Have Fun with Swings and Things • 20–21
**14.** Swings and Carriers • 22
**15.** Get Organized • 23

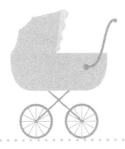

# Part 1

## Pre-Baby Preparation

Many mothers-to-be begin preparing for their babies the moment they find out they're pregnant. However, most women tend to focus on things like paint colors and baby clothing instead of more pressing issues. Of course, these are the fun aspects of having a baby, and you should take time to enjoy them. But much of what happens during the birth itself will impact your postpartum period. Early establishment of bigger decisions, like who will deliver your baby and where you will give birth, can help ensure a safe, satisfying delivery and postpartum experience.

# 1 Decide Who Will Be at the Birth

In addition to your partner, there will be at least a few other people present for the birth of your baby. One of the first decisions you will make will be with whom you will give birth. Will you choose a midwife or a doctor? What about a doula?

### Practitioners

Your first big choice is whether to deliver your baby under the care of a midwife or a doctor. Midwives are trained to assist with normal pregnancy, birth, and other well-woman care (birth control, annual exams, etc.). Many women with low-risk pregnancies enjoy the care of midwives while giving birth. Midwives may work in a hospital, birth center, or home-birth setting. Midwife training varies widely. Some midwives are nurses with master's degrees, some are certified by organizations like the North American Registry of Midwives (NARM), others have been trained at hospitals or birth centers, and many have a combination of training.

If you choose not to give birth with a midwife, you might prefer the help of a doctor. There are several different kinds of doctors available to you, including the family practitioner (FP) for low-risk women, the obstetrician/gynecologist (OB/GYN) for nearly every type of pregnancy, and the maternal fetal medicine (MFM) specialist for high-risk women. All of these doctors have attended medical school; what differs is the postgraduate residency course they completed. If you'd like to use your family practitioner, you must first be sure he delivers babies, as not every family practitioner incorporates birth into his practice.

### Doulas

*Doula* is a Greek word meaning "woman servant." Doulas are trained to help you and your family during the pregnancy, birth, and postpartum period using information, comfort measures, and other local resources. There are both birth and postpartum doulas. A birth doula specializes in helping families during late pregnancy, the birth, and the early postpartum days. A postpartum doula is trained to help the new family during the first few months postpartum.

## 2. Consider Important Delivery Details

Many women choose to give birth at home. Home birth is an option for low-risk women with qualified practitioners, doctors, or midwives. Today, many families are choosing home birth to have more control over their environment.

Birth centers offer a homelike environment for delivery, but you have a bit more support than you would at home. Doctors, midwives, or a combination may assist you. The emphasis in birth centers is on the low-risk woman who desires fewer interventions.

The majority of women choose to give birth in hospitals, as they are available for all women. Though many assume hospitals are the birth location best equipped to handle any kind of complication, this depends entirely on your individual situation.

### Create a Birth Plan

A birth plan is a basic plan, usually in the form of a document, created to help you, your partner, and your practitioner clarify your desires for the birth.

What a birth plan does is allow you and everyone supporting you to have a set of guidelines for how you'd like to approach your labor, birth, and postpartum experience.

## Take Childbirth Classes 3

Childbirth classes educate you and your partner about pregnancy, birth, the postpartum period, breastfeeding, and much more. What is taught in each class will depend on the educator, the theme of the class, and the location.

Take a class that covers everything, even details you don't think you'll need to know. For example, it is important that everyone understand the basics of cesarean surgery. While you may not think you will need a cesarean, once in labor it sometimes turns out to be the best birth method for women. It is equally important to learn techniques to help get you through labor without medication. That way, if you can't have medication or you prefer not to have it, you'll have the skills to help yourself during labor.

In addition to general childbirth classes, there are also specialty classes available. You might want to take an infant safety class or a vaginal birth after cesarean (VBAC) class. There are also classes on multiple births and breastfeeding. Specialty classes allow you to focus on a specific aspect that is important to you. Choose a class that has a great philosophy and an educator you like, and be sure it fits comfortably into your schedule.

## 4 Pack for the Hospital

Most mothers-to-be worry that they'll forget something when they pack for the hospital. Save yourself the stress! You likely won't forget anything important, and if you do, your partner, a family member, or a friend can easily go back and get it for you.

Here's a general list of essentials to include in your suitcase:

- Clothes to wear in labor
- Toiletries
- Massage tools, including lotions or oil
- Birth ball, if not provided
- Baby book, if you're keeping one
- Camera, batteries, and film or memory card
- Phone numbers of friends you'd like to call
- Nursing gown and bra
- Car seat for baby
- Going-home outfit for baby

When packing for labor and birth, pack two suitcases. One should be for labor and include anything that you would need during your labor and the first few hours after birth. The second suitcase can remain in the car until you're in your postpartum room. This should contain extra clothes, going-home outfits, and other items that aren't essential for labor.

## Decide When to Leave Work 5

Many women struggle to decide when to leave work before the baby is born. If you won't be working again for a few years, you might prefer to work right up until your due date. If you plan to return to work soon after you've recovered, you might appreciate more time to relax before the baby comes. Some women are simply worried about being at work when their water breaks. This is a personal decision each woman must make for herself.

**Your Due Date**

Your doctor will probably give you a due date, or a projected date for the birth. Don't make the mistake of counting on this being the exact date your baby will be born—it's really just a guess. Your baby can safely be born two weeks before or even two weeks after that date.

If your due date has been changed because of the size of your belly or the size of your baby, the new date may not be very accurate. Ultrasound due dates made after the first trimester are not very accurate either, as babies grow at different rates after that point. A due date is merely an estimate given to help you prepare for the baby.

## 6 Learn about Maternity Leave

Have a plan before you go speak with your boss about arranging maternity leave. Talk to your company's Human Resources Department or research your rights according to state or local regulations to educate yourself about the process. You might also consider talking to other new parents at work to see what types of job leave they had when their children were born.

Having an idea of the normal maternity leave process before you approach your boss will boost your confidence. This will also show your boss that you thoroughly understand your position. In showing her you care enough to do the research, your boss will see that you value your job and want to coordinate the best possible arrangement.

### Understand the Family Medical Leave Act (FMLA)

Federal law on family leave is called the Family Medical Leave Act (FMLA). You must work at a qualifying company, meaning your business has a certain number of employees, to take leave under this act. And your job must qualify, meaning you have worked full-time in your position for a year or more.

If you and your place of work meet the requirements, you can take up to twelve weeks of unpaid leave. This time is to be used for the birth of a baby, an adoption, or the caretaking of a sick immediate relative. The good news about the FMLA is that both you and your partner can use it, and in some cases both of you may choose to take some or all of this leave, while having your job status protected. Your partner's work may offer a paternity leave schedule, or he may use part of the FMLA time.

**Plan Thoroughly**

It is wise to negotiate your maternity leave by the time you are about seven months pregnant. This prepares you for any surprises in the pregnancy and allows you to relax, knowing that the negotiations are over. As the weeks before your due date start winding down, you should begin mentoring any coworkers who will be taking over your projects while you're out.

## 7 Budget for Baby

You may have heard people say that if you waited to have a baby until you could afford it, you'd never have children at all. While there is truth to this statement, there is also something to be said for being fiscally responsible in planning for your children. A new baby doesn't have to break the bank. The first step to success is knowing what expenses to expect.

**Pregnancy Expenses**

During pregnancy you will want some extra money for a variety of needs. Childbirth classes are one expense, and class fees vary widely depending on the class and its location. The fees for your doula may be covered by your insurance, but if not, you'll have that cost to consider.

In addition to paying the medical professionals for their services, you'll also have to buy a few basics during pregnancy, including maternity clothes. This can get expensive, as your shape and size will change fairly rapidly after the first trimester. However, a good way to save money is to buy secondhand maternity clothes, borrow maternity clothes from friends, or even make them yourself. An occasional pregnancy massage might also be on your list of expenses.

Unfortunately, you can't put your wallet away yet. There are several costs associated with the birth itself. A normal, uncomplicated vaginal birth costs about

$5,000, including prenatal care, without insurance. If you require anesthesia, such as an epidural, that will add another $1,200, and a cesarean costs about $3,000 extra. This total doesn't even include an additional nursery stay for your baby. However, there are a few ways to save money here. If you are low risk, a less expensive option for birth may be to use a midwife or birth center instead of a hospital. In addition to being more cost effective, these options tend to report higher patient satisfaction rates than hospitals do.

### Saving Up

If you plan to take a significant duration of unpaid leave from work, it's wise to accrue some savings to be used while you do not have income. Try to figure out your minimum budget. Decide how long you will be out of work and how much you will need to cover that time, then budget in that amount for the months remaining in your pregnancy. Remember to add about 10 percent extra for emergencies or an early birth.

If you will be leaving work for good, or if you'll be returning to work while your partner stays at home, it's a great idea to use those final months of income to build a nest egg. If you are able to bank vacation or sick days, do this too.

## 8 Get Help and Stock Up

As the birth approaches, you'll need to do some planning for how things will function once your little one arrives. You'll be focused on your new baby's needs, so who will take care of your other responsibilities? To keep everything running smoothly, you'll need to enlist the help of friends and family and keep your house stocked with the essentials at all times.

**Who Will Help?**

A postpartum doula is a valuable resource during late pregnancy and the first few weeks after the birth. Your doula might prepare meals for you, do the grocery shopping, or take care of the laundry. You can also ask friends and family for help with these things.

As the birth approaches and after the baby is born, friends and family will probably ask you the same question over and over again: "Can I help with anything?" Many people don't like to ask for help, but when you have a new baby at home, you could always use a little assistance. Prepare a list of things you need brought to you or need done around the house and keep it handy at all times. This way, when someone asks what she can do to help, you can offer her suggestions.

## Essential Items

Other than the usual supply of baby products, it's advisable to have two weeks worth of food and other essentials in the house at all times. Be sure to have plenty of toothpaste, paper towels, toilet paper, soap, and disposable dishes. You will not want to be standing over a sink washing dishes when you're only days away from your due date. Also stock up on nonperishable food items that can be used to make quick meals, such as pasta, rice, and canned soups. Preparing meals ahead of time and freezing them can also be helpful.

## 9 Choose a Pediatrician

Your pediatrician will be a very important part of your child's life, so put a lot of time and effort into your choice. Interview several pediatricians before selecting one. Whatever you do, don't just choose one from the phone book. You want to know and understand the pediatrician's philosophy. Does he value your opinions and concerns or see himself as the ultimate authority on child-rearing? You want someone who has your child's best interests at heart.

While the person's philosophy and demeanor are very important, you also need to be practical. The doctor's office should be close to your home or job, accept your insurance, and have office hours compatible with your schedule. It doesn't matter how fantastic the pediatrician is if you can't get to her office. You should also find out if there is a way to reach the pediatrician outside of his office hours in the event of a serious problem.

Chances are you won't find the "perfect" pediatrician, but this doesn't mean you shouldn't try. Don't lower your standards because you're tired of looking. The time and effort you put in now will be worth it in the end.

## Get a Car Seat  10

A car seat is a necessity (and a law) for a new baby. The problem is that there are so many styles of car seats that it's hard to determine which is best for you. The key to choosing a car seat will always be safety. Once you've found a safe, reliable car seat, good looks and fancy features are just perks.

**Infant Car Seats**

Infant car seats are designed to face backward in your car because it is easier for your baby to deal with the force of a crash with their weak neck muscles in this position. Infant car seats can be used until the weight specified for the particular carseat, usually around twenty pounds. In general, your baby is always safest in the rear seats of your car.

These types of car seats fit directly into the seat of your car and are strapped in with your car's regular seat belt (or Latch system, if your car has that option). Many infant car seats come with a "base." The base is strapped to the seat of your car with the seat belt, and you simply snap and unsnap the "carrier" portion of the car seat from the base. The baby is placed into the carrier, which has its own strap. This system allows you to take the baby in and out of the car without moving her too much (she can stay in the carrier).

## 10

### Toddler Car Seats

Toddler car seats face forward in your car and are used for babies who weigh more than twenty pounds. They are not usually used until your child is also one year of age and over twenty pounds. Most toddler car seats are designed to carry children until they are sixty to eighty pounds, though state laws vary on how old and how large your child has to be before he can leave a car seat.

A toddler car seat attaches to the car via the seat belt or Latch system in your car. It can be moved from car to car, but it is less convenient than the infant car seats. It does not double as a carrier. Speak to other parents about their toddler car seat choices before purchasing your own.

### Convertible Car Seats

The convertible car seat is supposed to be the best of both worlds. It can fit the smallest newborn in a rear-facing position and also converts to a forward-facing toddler seat. This also means you need only purchase one car seat as opposed to two car seats for your little one. However, there are complaints about the convertible car seats. The main complaint is that it can't be used as a carrier.

# Cribs, Bassinets, Cradles, and Co-sleepers 11

The crib is the classic place for a baby to sleep; in fact, you most likely slept in a crib as a baby. However, there are many options for places for your baby to sleep. Some are long-term options, while some are appropriate for only certain age ranges.

### Bassinets and Cradles

Bassinets and cradles are typically used for the first few months of your baby's life. Many families choose to use them to keep the baby closer to them while they sleep. These are smaller than the usual crib and don't allow the baby much room to move.

### Co-sleepers

A co-sleeper is great for your family if co-sleeping is what you would like to do. This product enables you to have your baby very close by, even in your bed with you, for ease of feeding in the night. A co-sleeper allows you to expand your bed, if the size of your bed was precluding you from considering co-sleeping.

Most co-sleepers come in portable and wooden varieties. The wooden ones can be converted into benches or desks as your child grows. The sleeping area in a co-sleeper is larger than a cradle or bassinet, but slightly smaller than a crib.

## 12 Invest in a Stroller

Strollers are the ultimate way to get your baby out and about. From getting exercise to simply strolling through the mall, a stroller can help you get out of the house and enjoy other activities. The key is choosing the right stroller for your lifestyle, or purchasing multiple strollers for different needs.

### Umbrella Strollers

Umbrella strollers are great for fast and furious shopping trips and quick strolls. They are very portable and also easy to store in the car, for those unexpected walks in the park on your way home from the grocery store.

While umbrella strollers are ultralightweight and easy to use, they can also be less sturdy. This is usually only a problem for toddlers or older children. Though they do come in sturdier versions, these tend to be a bit more expensive. Umbrella strollers can also be difficult to use with very young babies. Before your baby can hold his head up well, you will need a stroller in which your baby can lie down. Most umbrella strollers do not offer this option.

### Carriage Stroller

A carriage stroller is defined by the feature of allowing the baby to rest in a flat (or nearly flat) position. Also, the seat is supported by a frame that moves on four wheels. Large, set wheels allow for a smoother ride, and are recommended for mothers planning on lots of walking activities. Carriages set on smaller, swiveling wheels are better suited for quick turns and shopping. Carriage strollers also usually come with some sort of basket—either mesh or a wire rack—that is handy for hauling a diaper bag, or for shopping excursions.

### Double Strollers

Double strollers are a wonderful invention! They work great not only for moms with multiples, but also if you have an older child who wants to tag along. You may also consider a double stroller as an investment if you want more children in the future. Having the extra storage space is never a bad thing!

### Jogging Strollers

Jog strollers typically have large, bicycle-like wheels—one in the front and two in the back. They're useful for parents who are runners or joggers, and also on rougher terrain, such as unpaved paths. They can be pricey and large, but they're much easier to push and maneuver than a "regular" stroller when running or jogging. Consider your needs and research some of the many types available.

## 13 Have Fun with Swings and Things

Swings and other baby carriers can be great ways to help contain your baby for short periods of time. These carriers also offer a way to help soothe your baby, usually via movement. The main difference between the options is in the way the motion is created—by the baby or a battery.

### Swings

These infant seats are much like light car seats, suspended from a metal frame. A battery pack tends to power the motion for the swing. Swings come in many shapes and fashions.

Swings can be used to help soothe a baby to sleep, or as an easy way to entertain a tyke while you get a small task done. Just be sure not to leave your baby unattended in a swing.

### Bouncers

Babies like to bounce, and the motion is great for calming a crying or fussy baby. For this reason, there are several different bouncing gadgets on the market for babies.

Bouncer seats are usually cloth seats fitted to metal frames. Most of these seats include a safety strap that goes between your baby's legs and secures at the waist. Because these seats recline, they can be used even for small babies.

Bouncer seats are great for use with little ones. They can entertain and comfort at the same time. As your baby gets older and learns cause and effect, he'll begin to learn that when he moves, the chair bounces. Most models also have a toy bar across the front for extra fun, and some offer a "vibration" option that many babies find soothing.

**Stationary Jumpers**

This circular-based toy has a seat in the middle, and the seat rotates 360 degrees, giving your baby access to a variety of fun toys.

In the stationary jumper, your baby can stand and learn to use her leg muscles; however, some say that it isn't good to allow babies to bear weight on their legs before a certain age. Be sure to check with your pediatrician buying a stationary jumper.

**Johnny Jump-Ups**

These doorway jumpers hang from a doorway and allow your baby to jump up and down. This can be a great workout for an older baby, but again, there is the issue of weight bearing. For this reason, this product is not appropriate for smaller babies.

## 14 Slings and Carriers

Parents have busy lives and can't sit around holding their babies all day, even if they'd like to, so they need a way to hold their babies while getting other things done, from vacuuming the floor to talking on the phone.

### Slings

Slings are pieces of fabric that hold your baby on your body, distributing the weight from shoulder to hip. They can be used from the newborn period until your child weighs about thirty-five pounds. There are several different types of holds that can be used with the slings, depending on your preference and the baby's age.

### Front Packs

Front packs are simply backpacks for the front of your body. There are many varieties available, all with different systems of snaps and buttons to help you position your baby. Your baby can face either inward or outward.

The main complaint about these types of carriers is that they can be difficult to learn to use. However, once you learn to use them, they are a snap.

## Get Organized 15

Though your newborn baby will be quite tiny, she will have a ton of stuff! After the first couple of months, you may lose control over the products, toys, and clothing. Dressers, boxes, and closets may begin to overflow. Luckily, there are ways to get things organized. It just takes some time and diligence to sort it all out.

**Space Issues**

Look for portable or collapsible items for your baby. This might mean strollers that fold down to next to nothing, or a smaller, collapsible crib for your baby. It could also mean getting pieces of equipment that will last for a while or will serve more than one purpose, like a convertible car seat.

One way to keep organized is to select a place for each large item. You could keep the bouncer seat in your living room for when you need free hands to read mail. You can store the swing in the kitchen for times when you're cooking or cleaning.

As for the little objects that you have for baby, try baskets and bins. Use a container of some sort in each room. It should hold any small toys or books that you have for baby. As your baby gets older, use these containers to teach cleaning up. Simply show your baby that everything goes in the container when he's done playing.

**16.** Prepare for Your Birth • 26
**17.** Know What to Expect from Your Baby • 27
**18.** Will You Allow Visitors? • 28
**19.** Get What You Need at the Hospital • 29
**20.** How Will Your Body Look Afterward? • 30
**21.** How to Handle Postpartum Pain • 31–32
**22.** Soothe Specific Locations • 33
**23.** Prepare for Postpartum Emotions • 34
**24.** What is APGAR Scoring? • 35
**25.** Weighing, Measuring, and Blood Work • 36
**26.** Eye and Ear Screenings • 37
**27.** Breathing Difficulties • 38
**28.** What Is Meconium Staining? • 39
**29.** How to Handle Jaundice • 40
**30.** Bring Your Baby Home! • 41

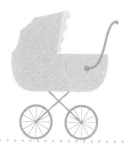

# Part 2

## The Birth and Your First Weeks as a Mom

Congratulations! You are about to be a new mom. Your pregnancy is nearly over and you have very few things left to do. Once you get set up for birth, whether it be at home, a birth center, or a hospital, you will hopefully be able to relax and enjoy the birth experience. You will spend your first few days as a mother relishing your time with your baby and getting accustomed to this new life. Your body and mind will be reeling from the experience, but this is perfectly normal and okay.

## 16 Prepare for Your Birth

Your birth experience is very important, as it will set the tone for your early days of mothering. In other words, the way you feel during the birth greatly affects the way you come to feel about your baby and your new role as a mother.

Having a vaginal birth is the most common experience. Yet within this one experience, there are many factors that will physically and emotionally influence your first few days as a mother.

If you have a vaginal birth without medication, you will probably feel like getting up to move around or go to the bathroom, sometimes within minutes of giving birth. This is perfectly fine, but stick close to someone in case you feel dizzy. If you have an epidural or other pain medication in labor, it will take time to wear off. You may not be able to walk around for several hours. This means you will require a catheter or bedpan to go to the bathroom. You will need help when you do get up, due to residual numbness or dizziness.

Whether or not your cesarean birth is planned, you will not be able to move for several hours. If you have had regional anesthesia such as an epidural or spinal, you may feel some numbness after the surgery. If you have had general anesthesia, you will not feel numb, but you will still be unable to walk around for some time.

## Know What to Expect from Your Baby

When she is born, your baby may cry, whimper, or be quiet, but none of these is a bad sign. The important thing is that the baby is breathing. Once this is ascertained, your baby should be handed to you right away. The best way to keep the baby warm is by holding her to your bare skin and covering her up with warm blankets. Even before the umbilical cord is clamped or cut, you can hold your baby as high on your chest as the cord will allow.

Your baby will probably feel a bit wet and potentially be tinged with blood. This is your blood—not the baby's blood. You or your partner can take a clean towel and dry the baby while your newborn gazes up at you (new babies can see best from a distance of about 8 to 12 inches) and listens to the sound of your heartbeat from the outside. Your baby will probably be wrinkled and may appear reddish or swollen. Don't worry if her head looks a bit misshapen. New babies' heads are designed to change shape as they fit through your pelvis. A normal, round head shape will develop as the skull hardens.

If your baby needs to be seen for emergency reasons or is taken to the neonatal intensive care unit (NICU) after birth, do not fear. This does not necessarily indicate tragedy, and you can still be with your baby in the NICU once you are both stable.

# 18 Will You Allow Visitors?

Everyone will be very anxious to meet your new baby. However, knowing there is an audience waiting outside your door can add to the stress of your labor and delivery. Consider telling everyone to wait at home, and promise to call at a certain point in labor or just after your little one has arrived.

### In the Birth Room

If you choose to have visitors during labor, it can be a nice distraction early on, but you'll probably find you don't want visitors once you get closer to delivery time. Know before you go into labor who you have invited and who you haven't. Don't be afraid to let your doula act as your bodyguard if you want to keep visitors at bay for a while.

To keep things comfortable and uncomplicated, go ahead and set a few ground rules. For instance, you can declare that anyone in the labor and birth room must be actively helping with the labor. If you don't allow casual observers in the room, then there won't be anyone staring at you while you pant through contractions. Being a part of the labor and helping out is one thing, but gawking in the corner and taking up space is completely another.

## Get What You Need at the Hospital 19

Chances are, getting what you need in terms of care at home or in a birth center will be fairly straightforward. At home you'll know where everything is and can easily ask someone to get an item for you. A birth center is a bit more difficult, but chances are you won't be there very long. However, you might have to negotiate a little to get what you need at a hospital.

Your birth plan should also contain a section that spells out your desires for the postpartum period. This can include details about visitors, getting help with breastfeeding, newborn care, and other areas of importance to you. Because hospitals are busy places with a lot of patients and not so many staff, you'll need to rely on this plan as your form of communication at certain points.

If this isn't successful or if your needs change, do not hesitate to tell your nurse or nurse's aide. The problem in a hospital is that you are on a list with others who also have needs. Therefore, having your own group of friends and family there to help you is a good idea. Having your partner and guests there to help most of the time will ease some of the burden on the nursing staff. This will also make things run more quickly and smoothly for you.

## 20 How Will Your Body Look Afterward?

You're probably worried about how your body will look after you give birth. What will your bottom look like, and will it ever be the same again? Will you have a scar from a repair or other surgery? Will your partner notice? These are all normal questions that every woman asks, and in most cases, things turn out just fine.

One of the first things you might think is how skinny you must be compared to those last days of your pregnancy! Your belly is now mostly deflated. Unfortunately, once you stand up and that loose skin falls southward, you'll have a soft pouch instead of a flat stomach. Don't worry, though—it takes some time for the skin to tighten back up.

When packing for the hospital or birth center, choose the outfit you will go home in wisely. The jeans you wore at your skinniest clearly aren't going to work, but you might not need a pair of pants from your ninth month of pregnancy either. Pack a comfortable mid-pregnancy outfit. You're not pregnant anymore, but your body definitely hasn't returned to its prepregnancy state yet either.

# How to Handle Postpartum Pain 21

Giving birth is taxing on your body, no matter how you do it. You will experience soreness from tensing your muscles during labor, aches and swelling at any surgery sites, and general symptoms of fatigue. Additionally, vaginal births and cesareans have different effects on the body. You may choose to take medication to relieve some of these aches and pains, but be sure to consult with your doctor before choosing any remedies, even over-the-counter and herbal products.

### Vaginal Birth

If you have a vaginal birth, your muscles will be sore from flexing and moving around while in labor. If stirrups are used, particularly for forceps or a vacuum delivery, then your legs may be sore around the hip area from hyperextension. Usually, a dose of ibuprofen will soothe the majority of muscle aches. For the first few days, you can take this by the clock—you won't want to wait for your pain to come back before taking another dose.

If your pain is severe, which is more likely if you have a forceps or vacuum birth or an episiotomy, there are other methods of pain relief available. Some are narcotics. These tend to make you feel a bit groggy but are very effective in relieving pain. They can also be used in combination with other over-the-counter medicines such as ibuprofen.

## 21

**Cesarean**

Your pain and soreness will be a bit different if you have a cesarean. If you have an epidural or spinal anesthesia, you can be given a medication called Duramorph during or after the administration of your anesthesia. This medication is administered in the same area as the epidural or spinal medications. It can provide pain relief for sixteen to twenty-four hours, without a numbing sensation. The most common side effect from this medication is itching. Be sure to ask your anesthetist about this—some people are allergic to this drug.

After the cesarean surgery is over and the numbness or general anesthesia wears off, ibuprofen can also be helpful to you. You will still feel the same uterine sensations as you would with a vaginal birth—these sensations indicate the healing of the uterus. The ibuprofen will ease afterpains—the pains from contractions that shrink the uterus. You may also use narcotics for this purpose. Narcotics for pain relief can be given orally, by injection, or in your IV line, and they tend to make you groggy. Be sure to ask what your doctor or midwife has ordered that you have after your surgery.

## Soothe Specific Locations  22

Though your whole body will likely be sore after giving birth, certain areas of your body will be especially tender. Primarily, your vagina will be sore, with or without tearing or stitches. If you do have stitches from a tear or episiotomy, you are more likely to have pain in this area. You may also have hemorrhoids from the pushing process.

If you have an epidural during childbirth, you may later have a sore spot in your back where the needle entered. A urinary catheter is frequently used in the epidural process, so you may have soreness or a numb feeling in your urethra as well, making it difficult to urinate.

Cold packs can help reduce swelling wherever you have it and particularly in your vaginal area. You can also use spray-on topical anesthetics to numb any painful areas. Ask your doctor or midwife which of these products is available and safe for your use.

Sitz baths are available to help promote healing and deal with the pain associated with childbirth. They can be done in the hospital or at home. These baths help keep your perineum clean while soothing the area. Ask your doctor or midwife about this option.

## 23 Prepare for Postpartum Emotions

Immediately after your baby is born, you will likely be exhausted but euphoric. You might not be able to take your eyes off your baby, even if there are doctors stitching you up and cleaning you off. You may cry out of joy over having your baby in your arms, out of relief that the labor is over, or for no particular reason at all.

Alternatively, you may feel not much of anything after your baby is born. Exhaustion may take over due to lack of sleep during late pregnancy. Physical symptoms may overshadow the joy of having a new baby—at least for a little while. However, postpartum depression is not common in the first few days. You'll probably just feel weary until your body has a chance to heal.

If you have a negative birth experience for whatever reason, it is okay to acknowledge this. It is also important that you express this to someone you trust who can validate your feelings. Just because you aren't pleased with your birth experience doesn't mean you don't love your baby. If you ignore these feelings, you can find yourself deep in postpartum depression.

# What Is APGAR Scoring? 24

The APGAR scoring system, named for its creator, Virginia Apgar, is a mnemonic device that covers five different ways of grading a baby at birth. This system is used to determine the baby's basic health status. APGAR stands for:

- Activity: muscle tone
- Pulse: heartbeats per minute
- Grimace: reflex irritability
- Appearance: skin color
- Respiration: absence or presence of breath

Your baby is given a score of 0, 1, or 2 for each category, with 10 being a perfect score. A score of 7 to 10 is considered normal, 4 to 7 might call for resuscitative action, and 3 or below requires immediate resuscitation. Your baby will be graded one minute after birth and again at five minutes. If your baby is having a rough time getting started, you will also have a third score after ten minutes. This scoring usually goes unnoticed by parents. While you are consumed with the emotion of new motherhood, a nurse or midwife will be keeping a sharp eye on your baby for labored breathing or other signs of stress.

## 25 Weighing, Measuring, and Blood Work

You'll probably be very excited to know how much your baby weighs and measures. These numbers stick in most mothers' heads forever. Just keep in mind that these measurements do not indicate the health or ultimate body type your child will have. A seven-pound baby can be just as healthy as a nine-pound baby, and one that measures twenty-two inches will not necessarily grow to be taller than a baby born at nineteen inches.

Weighing and measuring is usually done in the first couple of hours of life, but it doesn't need to happen right away. After you have spent some time nursing and cuddling with your baby, you can declare that she's ready to be measured.

You may also be asked to permit a routine blood screening for metabolic disorders such as phenylketonuria, thyroid issues, sickle cell, and other problems. This is usually done with a heel stick. Feel free to hold or nurse your baby during the procedure to comfort him and ease any pain. Be sure your baby is at least forty-eight hours old when blood screening is done. If performed prior to this time, the results may be invalid and the screening must be repeated.

## Eye and Ear Screenings 26

Your state law may mandate eye medication following the birth. Check with your local government to find out what the laws are in your community. The eye ointment is administered to prevent blindness in your baby in case you have an untreated sexually transmitted infection (STI). Even if eye medication is mandated, you can still choose when it's done and what medication is used. For example, erythromycin is much gentler than the silver nitrate alternative. Many moms also wait for an hour or two before using the medication because it can cause blurry vision. This may be a bit annoying for your newborn but not harmful.

Where the ears are concerned, many states now require that hearing screenings be done on newborns. These screenings work best when your baby is asleep. So, during the night, a nurse may tap on your door and ask for the baby. Feel free to send the baby with your partner or bring him yourself for this brief test. Bringing the baby ensures that he will return to your room with you as soon as the test is complete.

## 27 Breathing Difficulties

Some babies will have breathing difficulties at birth. If your baby is born early or via cesarean section, she will be more likely to have these problems. Usually, the doctor or midwife can facilitate breathing by rubbing the baby's skin, possibly giving her oxygen. This can be done in any birth setting.

All practitioners are also trained to provide CPR on your newborn, if needed. Long-term ventilation and other breathing treatments may be available only at a Level II or III hospital setting. These measures are the least likely to be needed.

# What Is Meconium Staining?

Once your water breaks, it may become apparent that your baby has passed his first bowel movement while still inside your body. This is called meconium staining. Meconium is seen in cases where the baby is overdue, stressed, or both. If your practitioner sees meconium, she is likely to listen to the baby more frequently during labor to ensure he is not stressed.

As your baby is born, he will be suctioned before he can breathe or scream. This is done to prevent him from inhaling the meconium. Because meconium is thick and tarlike, it can make it difficult for a newborn to expand his lungs. So, removing it prior to screaming or breathing is important.

In the case of meconium staining, you may have to wait a few minutes before your baby is handed to you. Someone may perform deeper suctioning once the baby is completely free of the birth canal, also to prevent inhalation of meconium. Some babies will still inhale the meconium despite all efforts to prevent this. If your baby does this, he may need further tests, including X-rays. In some cases, a baby will also need to stay in the NICU. Your doctor will explain more about this in the unlikely event that it becomes necessary.

## 29 How to Handle Jaundice

Jaundice is the collection of bilirubin in the blood. This can be discovered through a blood test, but more likely it will be discovered because a baby has turned a shade of yellow. This usually doesn't happen until the first few days after birth.

The best way to get rid of the bilirubin is to encourage as much breastfeeding as possible. Breast milk, particularly the colostrum it contains during the first few days, acts as a natural laxative, helping your baby to pass the bilirubin. Exposure to natural light through a window can also help.

Extreme cases of jaundice are rare. They are usually treated by breastfeeding and light therapy. Light therapy is usually done by using light blankets. A couple of days are all that is needed to clear up the condition.

# Bring Your Baby Home! 30

Finally, you've survived pregnancy, labor, and delivery, and your baby has arrived! Now it's time to take your new bundle of joy home. Bringing your new baby home for the first time is a thrilling and daunting experience. When you last left your home, there were only two of you; now you have a family of three.

In addition to a car seat, remember to bring a blanket or other device to help shield your baby from the rain or sun. You may want to ride in the backseat with your baby during the first car trip or two to watch and comfort her. You may find that you see the world differently once your baby is riding in your car. Suddenly it may seem like every car is pointed directly at yours and every pothole is a deep abyss waiting to swallow her up. These initial fears are normal and will fade in time.

The key to surviving the first days of new motherhood is to be prepared, flexible, and confident. Also, don't be afraid to go after whatever you need. If you need help, ask for it. Be sure to get your questions answered as soon as they come up. And most importantly, enjoy yourself!

**31.** Breastfeed If Possible • 44
**32.** Artificial Baby Milk (ABM), or Formula • 45
**33.** Bath Time! • 46
**34.** Make Diaper Decisions • 47–48
**35.** What Is Infant Potty Training? • 49
**36.** Hold Your Baby • 50
**37.** How to Handle Crying • 51
**38.** Learn the Newborn Sleep Basics • 52
**39.** Consider Co-sleeping • 53
**40.** Crib Sleeping • 54
**41.** Taking Your Baby Out of the House • 55
**42.** Develop a Routine • 56
**43.** Talk to Your Baby • 57
**44.** Read to Your Baby • 58
**45.** Incorporate Music into Your Life • 59

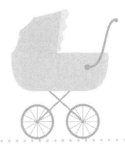

# Part 3

## Baby Care Basics

Transitioning to parenthood can be overwhelming. Suddenly, you have a tiny, helpless baby to feed, clean, clothe, and care for. It's a daunting task! However, if you helped take care of younger siblings while growing up, or did some babysitting when you were a teenager, these experiences will give you a good starting point for raising your own child. If you didn't have either of these experiences, don't panic. Your baby and your instincts will guide you in your new role.

## 31 Breastfeed If Possible

Breastfeeding is the natural choice for feeding your baby. Your body knows what to do, as does your baby. Even so, you need to learn about breastfeeding. Prenatal classes will teach you basic techniques, as well as explain how breastfeeding benefits both you and your baby. Not only will you learn to read your baby's hunger cues, but you will also learn different nursing positions and how to tell if your baby is getting enough milk.

If you are having difficulties, be sure to talk to other moms who have successfully nursed. You can also get help from a local lactation consultant or through La Leche League International, an organization providing information and encouragement to breastfeeding mothers.

Breastfeeding can be a lot easier for mom than bottle-feeding pumped breast milk or artificial baby milk. Coming from the breast, milk is always available and at the right temperature. Support, information, and patience are all you need to create a successful breastfeeding relationship with your baby.

## Artificial Baby Milk (ABM), or Formula

If you make the decision to feed your baby ABM (usually called formula), you may also need to take a class on how to properly feed your baby formula using a bottle. The bottle and the formula you choose will largely depend on what your pediatrician or hospital provides, as it can be stressful for the baby if you switch to a different milk. However, you may need to switch if the original choice doesn't meet your baby's needs or gives him gas. Be sure to follow the instructions on the formula can.

You will need to choose a premade, condensed, or powdered formula. There is not really a difference for your baby, but there may be variations in cost and how long each will stay fresh in your home. You may need to heat the formula using boiling water or a bottle warmer. Do not use a microwave.

While your baby eats, watch for indications that she's getting full. Just because there's still milk in the bottle doesn't mean you should force your baby to finish; this won't make her sleep longer and it may make her ill. Take your time when feeding your baby. Make eye contact with her, talk to her, and switch sides at least once during each feeding, to encourage brain development.

## 33 Bath Time!

While infants don't get dirty the way young children do, they do require occasional baths to keep their skin healthy. Daily baths are not needed until your baby starts crawling on the floor. A bath two or three times a week, in addition to thorough cleansing after feedings and changes, is sufficient until your baby is mobile.

### Bathe with Your Baby

Bathing with your little one is a great way to calm a baby who especially dislikes or fears baths. You can nurse the baby while in the tub to further distract him and passively get him used to the feel of the water; however, be aware that many newborns will have a bowel movement almost immediately after nursing.

### In the Tub and in the sink

There are several tubs for new babies on the market—some much more elaborate than others. The problem with using them in the bathtub is that you'll probably have to kneel and lean over to reach your baby.

Bathing your newborn in the sink is often simpler and safer because you can stand up and do it without having to lean over the tub.

## Make Diaper Decisions  34

As a new parent, you will spend a good portion of your day changing diapers. The average newborn goes through about eight to ten diapers every day. That's approximately seventy diapers in your first week alone. Gaining knowledge about diapering before you're faced with this nearly constant task can be very helpful.

**Cloth Diapers**

Many moms say that they use cloth diapers for a variety of reasons, especially to reduce rashes and to address environmental concerns. Whatever your reasons for choosing cloth diapers, be sure to research the pricing and find a good deal for quality equipment.

Cloth diapers have changed significantly since your mother or grandmother used them. Nowadays, there is no need for diaper pins or plastic pants. Modern diapers and diaper covers are mostly made of waterproof, breathable material and have Velcro closures. There are also diaper services that provide you with the diapers, clean them, and return them to you. However, you can still purchase the cloth diapers yourself and do it on your own the old-fashioned way.

### Diaper Services

One way to make cloth diapering a little more manageable is to use a diaper service. For slightly more money and depending on your location, you can have clean diapers delivered right to your door.

Usually a diaper service will give you seventy diapers and a pail. You simply put the dirty diapers in the pail and once a week on a specified day they will take the dirty diapers and give you clean ones. This option is more expensive than buying and cleaning the diapers yourself, but it saves you the hassle of washing upward of seventy diapers every week.

### Disposable Diapers

If you're not too thrilled about the cloth-diaper option, you can turn to the disposable-diaper alternative. Just as cloth diapers have developed over the years, disposable diapers have also become more comfortable for babies and manageable for parents.

Disposable diapers are made of paper and are used only once before being discarded. Don't let the word *paper* here worry you—these diapers are totally waterproof. In fact, disposable diaper materials have changed to help keep your baby dry and clean feeling, even while wearing the dirtiest diaper.

## What Is Infant Potty Training?

No, this is not a typo—infant potty training (IPT) is a real method used by some parents instead of diapers. Elimination communication is not a new idea, but it is making a comeback. To "potty train" your infant, you must learn to watch for cues from your baby that he needs to go to the bathroom. These cues are just as noticeable as those indicating hunger, tiredness, and any other strong sensation your baby might feel. When you realize that your little one has to go, you simply hold a bucket or other receptacle under the baby (or hold him over the toilet) while he relieves himself. Supporters of this method tout its many benefits; for instance, you save money and protect the environment by not buying or throwing away diapers. Additionally, it is suggested that teaching babies to eliminate in diapers and then potty training a couple of years later only confuses children. If you're interested in learning more about IPT, there are several books and websites that offer details, products, and advice.

## 36 Hold Your Baby

You will spend lots of time holding your baby—to comfort her, to move her from one place to another, and just to enjoy being close to her. This is one of the ways you and your partner bond with your baby. Go ahead and let friends and family hold your baby as well. It's important that she come to know all the people in her life from an early age.

### Skin-to-Skin Contact

Your baby will likely be given to you to hold close to your body as soon as he is born. This is because skin-to-skin contact with you has important benefits, including warming her and helping her to regulate her breathing. However, this contact is not only important on the day of birth; its value holds true throughout infancy. So, take some time each day to hold your baby close to your bare skin during those first few months. Your baby will enjoy the warmth of your body and the sound of your heartbeat, and you'll love the soft sensation of contact with your baby.

## How to Handle Crying

It's important to remember that babies cry—it's just a fact of life. Without verbal abilities, your infant doesn't have too many options when it comes to getting your attention. Crying doesn't necessarily mean that your baby is hurt, and it doesn't mean you've done something wrong. Your baby will cry for many reasons. The cause could be physical (he's hungry, tired, in pain, or wet/dirty) or emotional (he's frustrated, scared, lonely, overstimulated, or bored).

When your baby cries, try not to get frustrated. Instead, be a problem solver. Assess the situation by asking yourself questions. Could your baby be hungry? Does he need to be changed? Might he be tired? In some cases your baby will be asking you for a change of environment. For instance, if he is in a swing, moving him to a calmer place—like a blanket on the floor—might help him relax.

Unfortunately, your baby will sometimes cry for seemingly no reason at all. You might try every trick in the book, but to no avail. This can be extremely frustrating for both you and your baby. When this happens, hand your baby off to someone else, if possible. This will allow you to calm down and might even distract the baby from his carrying on. If there is no one else around, put your little one someplace safe, like in his car seat on the floor, and regain your composure.

## 38 Learn the Newborn Sleep Basics

Newborn babies sleep about twelve to eighteen hours a day during the first month of life. Generally, periods of wakefulness become longer as they get older. The problem with this is that most babies will not sleep for long stretches of time—especially at first—preventing you from getting sufficient sleep. But as time goes on, your baby will sleep longer and longer, and so will you.

Partially determining how well your baby sleeps will be the environment in which she sleeps. If you suspect your baby is not getting enough sleep, consider her environment. Do you leave the lights on? Does your baby share a room with a sibling who snores loudly? Is the room temperature comfortable? These and other details play a major role in how well your baby sleeps at night.

Sleeping through the night is really only possible when your baby is neurologically ready. It cannot be forced by feeding your baby cereal, letting your baby cry, or any other rumored "cure." Always be skeptical when presented with surefire methods to make your baby sleep through the night.

## Consider Co-sleeping 39

Co-sleeping, also called "sleep sharing" or "the family bed," simply means having your baby in bed with you. It is beneficial for you as well as your baby and will not cause your baby to become dependent on you to sleep. Your baby will eventually leave your bed when you are both ready.

Sharing sleep with your baby is a natural extension of baby care, particularly during the first months of life. Sleeping with your baby will make breastfeeding at night very simple, as there is no need to get out of bed, turn on lights, and sit up to feed your baby. This will probably help both of you get more sleep as well.

Many babies sleep better when comforted by the presence of their parents. It has also been shown in some studies that babies who sleep with their parents are less likely to have problems with sudden infant death syndrome (SIDS). Researchers speculate this is because the baby falls into your sleep patterns.

The rules for co-sleeping are simple: Don't sleep on a water bed. Don't be crowded in bed—use a queen- or king-sized bed if possible. Don't go to bed intoxicated or on pain medication. And end co-sleeping when you feel your child is naturally ready to sleep alone.

## 40 Crib Sleeping

You may decide that a crib is the best place for your baby to sleep. To prevent injury to your baby, be sure to choose a crib that meets the most current safety standards. This includes ensuring that the crib has slats that are close enough together, the crib does not contain toxic paint or other materials, and the mattress is of safe firmness. Don't be seduced by cute crib toys and decorations. It is best for the baby to sleep with nothing but a small, lightweight blanket—or, even better, a sleepsack. This means no toys, bumpers, pillows, or other items should be in the crib with her.

You'll find many schools of thought about how to get your baby used to sleeping in a crib. Here's one method to consider: hold or rock your baby until she is very sleepy or in a light stage of sleep before laying her down in the crib. If your baby wakes up as soon as you move her, you may need to wait until she is in a deeper sleep stage. Remember that even if the baby is not sleeping in your bed, or maybe not even in your room, you still need to be physically responsive to her at any time of night. Make sure she is relatively close by or use a monitor so you can hear any sounds of distress.

## Taking Your Baby Out of the House    41

Most new parents worry about taking a new baby out of the house. They don't want to expose their child to unknown dangers, especially while driving in the car. To get accustomed to leaving the house with the baby, start with short trips first. As you build your confidence, longer trips will come naturally.

In addition to the act of taking the baby into the outside world, the amount of supplies you need to take with you can be very daunting. You will need to tote around quite a few things in your diaper bag. These may include several changes of clothes, a blanket, a few toys, several diapers, wipes, medications, and much more. If you regularly carry a diaper bag, be sure to restock it as soon as you come home. This will ensure you're always ready to go. You should also put your diaper bag near the door, making it easy to grab on your way out.

## 42 Develop a Routine

Though you're used to operating by the time on the clock, your baby operates on a natural, instinctive schedule. His tiny tummy can't go as long without eating, and your baby requires frequent sleep for short periods of time. It will take time to join this way of life with your own, but it will happen.

You should not be rigid about when your baby does something and for how long. Follow the cues your baby sends you to show when he is satisfied and when he needs something. As your baby begins to disengage and appear sleepy, try putting him down for a nap. If your baby is alert and interacting with you, sing and play to entertain him. Your baby will let you know what he needs from you. Your only challenge is learning to read his signs and signals.

Don't let the thought of caring for your new baby overwhelm you. Remember that everyone makes mistakes, and these mistakes are rarely disastrous. Try out different techniques until you find what works best for you. And no matter how busy you get or how hectic life becomes, always take time to enjoy the experience of being a parent.

## Talk to Your Baby   43

One of the best ways to teach your baby is to talk to her. Through hearing your voice, she will learn a lot about language and other rhythmic patterns in speech far before she can use these skills herself. She will also pick up tone and emotion in your voice.

The question is, what do you have to talk about with a newborn? If she can't respond, how can you make effective conversation? For many new parents, talking to their babies does not come easily at first. To ease into it, just try giving her a rundown of her daily activities: "It's bath time! Let's get you undressed. First we take off your shirt. Now it's time for your diaper. Feel the warm water? Do you like the water?"

Over time, the conversations will become more natural and your baby will seem more and more interested in the words you say. Your baby will learn to understand not only patterns of speech, but schedules as well. Soon she'll associate all your babbling about getting undressed with bath time.

## 44 Read to Your Baby

You may think your baby won't develop any reading skills until she enters school, but this is actually not the case. Studies suggest that reading to your infant after she's born are great ways to interact with and teach your baby.

### Reading Books

Select a couple of books with big, bright pictures and very few words to start.

With a very young baby, simply sit him on your lap. Open the book and rest it on your knees at a comfortable viewing height and distance for your baby. As your baby ages, let him help you turn the pages. He will enjoy the feel of the pages, as well as any special textures that are included in the book.

In the latter half of your baby's first year, he may start "reading" to you. The words he says may be mostly unintelligible, and the stories he tells may not make any sense at all, but this is a very healthy form of self-expression. Plus, he will take great pride in "reading" to you. He will want to hold the books and turn the pages the way you do when you read to him.

## Incorporate Music into Your Life 45

Music, specifically classical music, is thought to be a great source of stimulation for babies. Some studies have shown that infants exposed to classical music develop into smarter children than those who do not hear the classics early on in life. Other studies dispute this finding. Of course, this doesn't mean that other music genres won't be beneficial to your baby. Any type of music will develop her sense of auditory recognition.

There is no specific music regimen guaranteed to boost your baby's intelligence. While classical music is often touted as the key to success, you can choose a collection of different genres to stimulate your baby. Play classical music during calm times, like before naps, and play more lively tunes with beats during playtimes.

There are a few musical activities you might consider trying out with your baby. Some schools, libraries, or other organizations might offer sing-along programs that you can attend with your baby. These programs allow you to meet other members of the community, sing and play simple instruments with your baby, and generally have a lot of fun.

**46.** What to Eat Right after the Birth • 62
**47.** Make a Postpartum Nutrition Plan • 63
**48.** Keep It Simple • 64
**49.** How Much Do Babies Eat? • 65
**50.** Breastfeeding 101 • 66
**51.** Breastfeeding Multiples • 67
**52.** Choose the Right Breast Pump • 68
**53.** Pumping Tips • 69
**54.** What to Do about Leaking Breasts • 70
**55.** Bottle-feeding 101 • 71
**56.** What Kind of Bottle Should You Use? • 72
**57.** Bottle-feeding Multiples • 73
**58.** When to Wean • 74–75
**59.** Starting Solids • 76
**60.** Feeding Your Baby from the Table • 77

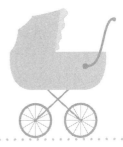

# Part 4

## Nutrition for the Family

Nutrition is a very important issue for new mothers and their babies. You need certain nutrients to heal after birth, and your baby needs the proper nutrition to grow into a healthy child. There are also different methods of feeding your baby to consider. Will you breastfeed or bottle-feed? When will you start feeding solid foods to your baby? Here you'll find all the information you need to make these decisions.

## 46 What to Eat Right after the Birth

During the postpartum period, your body is in the process of healing from pregnancy and birth. Continuing the great habits you formed while pregnant will contribute to keeping you healthy and strong during the first few months after birth.

One of the first things many new mothers want immediately after birth is food. The hard work of labor and delivery will likely leave you ravenous. Unfortunately, most labor and birth units don't have very appetizing options available. You may be offered only gelatin, pudding, or broth at first. If you're lucky, you'll get a sandwich. It's better to send a family member out for food that will actually satisfy your hunger. However, if you have a cesarean, you may not be able to eat at first and might be put on a clear-liquid diet for twelve to twenty-four hours.

Once you're out of the delivery room and in the regular postpartum unit, meals will be served regularly. Despite the countless jokes about hospital food, many hospitals go to great lengths to serve nutritious, delicious meals. Many times you will be given a couple of choices from a menu for the duration of your stay. If you have any special dietary needs or concerns, you will want to talk to your doctor or midwife as well as your nutritionist at the hospital prior to birth.

## Make a Postpartum Nutrition Plan 47

It's a good idea to discuss your postpartum diet with a nutritionist. If there is no nutritionist available to you at the hospital or birth center, consider speaking with the nutritionist from your practitioner's office. A basic understanding of good postpartum nutrition will be very helpful as you take care of yourself and your growing family.

It will be important to get a balanced diet, including lots of protein, fruits and vegetables, and carbohydrates.

# 48 Keep It Simple

The easiest way to ensure your family is fed well is to plan ahead. One specific thing you can do is choose four or five meals to make every week. You don't always have to eat the same thing on the same day, but keeping your options simple and defined will help you stay in control.

### Cook Ahead

There are a couple of different ways to cook ahead, and either can work wonderfully for a family. You can either double the recipe each time you cook and freeze half for another day, or select a single cooking day each month and prepare large enough quantities to last for the next few weeks. Both of these options make it easier for a family to eat nutritious, home-cooked meals every day.

### Cook Simply

The two things you must balance as a new mother are nutrition and time. You simply won't have the time to prepare such elaborate meals. However, this doesn't mean you have to sacrifice flavor. Many simple meals can be quite delicious, even if they didn't take forever to make. Don't fall into the trap of equating good food with lots of work. Instead, use a few simple tricks to make great food, like casseroles and slow-cooked meals, with ease.

# How Much Do Babies Eat?

If there's one thing you'll be doing more than anything else during the first months of motherhood, it's feeding the baby. However, the truth is that new babies don't really eat a lot—they just eat very often. Newborns have very tiny stomachs. To help you visualize how much milk they need, keep this in mind: A newborn's stomach is the size of a marble. After ten days, it grows to the size of a shooter marble. Even at three months it's only the size of a golf ball. Any myths you hear about new babies consuming gallons of milk in one feeding are wild exaggerations.

Learning to feed your baby may come naturally or it may be challenging, but with a little help and support, you will come to master it. All you have to do is ask for help. Be sure to see the lactation consultant at the hospital, or one who is connected with your practitioner.

## 50 Breastfeeding 101

Feeding your baby is obviously a huge part of the first year. Breast milk is a species-specific milk, meaning it is made by a human specifically for a human baby. It is the best food you can give your baby. Though your breast milk is pretty much all ready for your baby as is (and your baby is ready for your breast milk), there are certain things you can do to make breastfeeding go even more smoothly.

The best advice for a breastfeeding mother is to relax. Your baby will let you know how much milk she needs and when she's ready for it. Also, your breasts are designed to follow your baby's lead. After the first few days of life, look for five to six wet diapers a day and two to three bowel movements. The bowel movements may lessen as your baby ages. These are the signs of a baby who is getting enough to eat.

Your baby will pull away from the breast when she is ready to do so. Likewise, there is no set minimum amount of time that should pass between feedings. Your baby will give you hunger cues and it's best not to ignore them or make her wait.

You don't necessarily have to feed from both breasts at each feeding. Some babies will fill themselves at one breast. You should offer the second breast and see how your baby reacts. If she doesn't want to nurse right then, begin the next feeding with the fullest breast when she is ready.

# Breastfeeding Multiples 51

Your body knows how many babies you give birth to. In response, it will create enough milk to feed all of your babies. In fact, your body will usually provide more milk than one baby needs, even when you only have one. This is to ensure that the baby is never left hungry.

Take a breastfeeding class during your pregnancy. Find other mothers of multiples who have successfully breastfed. Talk to a lactation consultant during your hospital stay. Ask her for support in feeding your babies. They will be able to offer great positioning advice as well as other tips on feeding multiple babies.

Once you get past the hurdle of figuring out how to breastfeed and accommodating each baby's personality, it gets much easier. Remember, breastfeeding may be uncomfortable at first, but any discomfort should subside after the first few days, and any pain should never be extreme or long lasting.

## 52 Choose the Right Breast Pump

There will be times when you need to be away from your baby and you'll need to extract and collect your milk, either through the use of a breast pump or by hand expression. There are a few intricacies to take into account when it comes to pumps, including different sizes and styles.

### Big Pumps

The more often you intend to use your breast pump and the more milk you need to extract, the more likely you are to need an electric pump. These can be hospital grade, meaning the motor is designed to help you pump lots of milk at one time, fairly quickly.

There are also single-user electric pumps available for purchase. These are a good option for women returning to work or those who need to express a lot of milk at once.

### Small Pumps

Smaller breast pumps are usually hand or battery operated. These smaller pumps are designed for occasional use. They are perfect for a single replacement feeding every couple of days, but it would be difficult to use these on a daily basis for very long.

## Pumping Tips 53

It may take you a while to get the hang of pumping. Remember, your baby is the expert at extracting milk from your breasts—pumps will be only second best. Consider practice pumping by nursing your baby on one breast while simultaneously pumping the other (you may need your partner to help you coordinate that!). This lets your baby help regulate the hormones of letdown and increase your milk supply at the same time.

If you're pumping while you're away from your baby, try to think of your baby. Some mothers bring pictures of their babies with them to look at while they pump. Others just try to close their eyes and relax while thinking of their baby's smile. Thoughts of your baby will help stimulate milk production.

In addition to the pump itself, there are other products you can buy to make pumping easier. For one, you can find hands-free pumping bras for sale at many locations. These bras allow you to hook up the pump and keep your hands free for other tasks. If you're returning to work, you might want to invest in a breast pump microwave sterilizer. You simply rinse out the parts and put them in this round device with some water on the bottom. It takes only five minutes in the microwave to sterilize your pump.

## 54. What to Do about Leaking Breasts

Right after your baby is born, your breasts produce a premilk substance called colostrum. Colostrum is rich in antibodies and helps your baby pass his first stool, called meconium. Colostrum comes in very minute quantities, because your baby needs only a tiny bit. In the first few days after birth, your breasts will begin to produce what is called mature milk.

At first your body will seem to produce enough milk for the whole neighborhood. This is because your body is trying to satisfy even the heartiest appetite. This quantity can support more than one baby if you give birth to multiples. Because of the extra quantity, you may notice that milk leaks from one breast when your baby is nursing on the other side, or from both breasts when your baby cries. (Leaking when your baby cries is a conditioned response to your baby's needs, which lessens drastically as your baby gets older.) Sometimes you will leak if your breasts are overfull, showing you that your baby needs to eat.

The easiest way to deal with leaking breasts is to wear breast pads. It's important to ensure that the breast pads you select are not backed with plastic. You need breathable material to help prevent nipple soreness and potential yeast infection. These pads simply fit inside your bra. You can buy disposable pads for one-time use. There are also thick cotton washable pads available for repeated use.

## Bottle-feeding 101

Bottle-feeding is not as simple as popping a bottle in your baby's mouth. There are many different types of bottles and nipples, as well as some safety information you should know before feeding your baby with a bottle. With a little time and research, you can have a safe and satisfying bottle-feeding experience.

One thing to remember about bottle-feeding is that you must hold your baby while you feed him. You should hold your baby close and talk to him while feeding, as well as switch sides and arms during feedings.

Holding the baby close and talking to him makes the experience feel safe and comfortable. Don't consider feeding something you have to do to keep your baby alive; it's also a time to bond with your baby. Make sure everyone who feeds your baby a bottle understands how you feel about feedings and does what's necessary to keep the experience calm and comforting.

## 56 What Kind of Bottle Should You Use?

There are many types of bottles. Some are plastic; some are glass. Some are disposable and some are reusable. The types of bottles that work best for you will depend on several factors. How often do you intend to use a bottle? Who will be feeding your baby with a bottle? Will you be feeding stored breast milk in the bottle? How will you wash the bottles?

Disposable bottles can cost more in the long run and are worse for the environment than reusable alternatives. However, disposables are great for traveling, as you won't have to carry used bottles with you until they can be washed. Regular reusable bottles require washing and sterilizing. They also take up a lot of room. However, they are more cost effective and kinder to the environment than disposable varieties are.

Except for disposable bottles, all bottles must be washed out. You will need some special tools to help you accomplish this task. A bottle brush is a must, as is a nipple brush. These tools thoroughly remove bits of food that remain after rinsing.

If you hand-wash your bottles, you may wish to invest in a drying rack to allow the bottles to air-dry. To sterilize your bottles, you can boil them in water, sterilize them using a special sterilizing pot made for this purpose, or use a microwave sterilizer. Putting bottles in the dishwasher (after an initial rinse) is a great option, as it will both wash and sterilize your bottles.

## Bottle-feeding Multiples 57

Some multiples will need supplementation by alternative means. This can be by finger-feeding, cup-feeding, syringe-feeding, or even bottle-feeding. However, nursing moms (especially those with multiples) should try to avoid bottle-feeding until their milk supply is well established. If any of your babies is having trouble latching on, consider avoiding bottles and using alternative methods of feeding your baby. This will help prevent additional problems with a breastfeeding latch.

You may wish to alternate feedings of your multiples, particularly when the number of babies outnumbers the number of breasts available.

Multiple bottles or cups can be a pain to keep clean. Be sure to enlist help in the washing, drying, and sterilizing of these items. Microwavable sterilizers can be very handy, and they decrease the need for huge numbers of feeding accessories. They are also good for sterilizing toys, breast pump parts, and other baby items.

If you use artificial baby milk, it is possible to mix or make up what you need only once a day. Many families do this in pitchers, stored in the refrigerator. Be sure to check labels for how to mix formula, particularly when making it in larger quantities.

## 58 When to Wean

Weaning from the breast and weaning from the bottle are two different things. They can occur at different times and may be met with different attitudes. Whether you wean your baby suddenly or gradually is a matter of choice, but don't be surprised if your baby seems opposed to the idea.

**Weaning from the Bottle**

By the age of one year, most babies should not be using a bottle; a cup will be sufficient for drinking. Your child may fight you on this, but it needs to happen. Choose to quit using bottles all at once or remove them gradually. For the cold turkey option, you might pick a certain day to say bye-bye to the bottle. Perform some sort of ceremony to present weaning from the bottle in a positive light. Tell your baby what a big boy he is now that he drinks from a cup. There may still be tears shed over losing the bottle, but your baby will adapt to the change in time.

If you choose to gradually wean your baby off the bottle, you may decide to start by removing the bottle from one meal a day. This may be easier in the daytime, as most toddlers prefer the bottle early in the morning and at bedtime. Remember, the action of sucking is comforting to babies. To wean gradually, just continue to remove the bottle from meals one at a time until the baby is no longer using the bottle at all.

## Weaning from the Breast

Weaning from the breast can be led by the baby or by the mother. Around one year of age, if the mother wishes to wean, she will start cutting out one feeding a week. Generally, a one-year-old nurses only two or three times a day in short bursts, so feedings will decrease relatively rapidly at this rate.

Another approach to mother-led weaning is to discontinue offering the breast to the baby. If you normally wake up and immediately nurse your baby, try a new ritual instead. If the baby forgets he usually nurses during this time, don't remind him. However, if he shows he wants to nurse, go ahead and breastfeed. When he's ready, he'll stop asking for the breast.

Weaning from the breast is usually easier than weaning from a bottle because it can be replaced with the cuddling and loving associated with nursing. Most children will eventually wean themselves. The key here is that as long as mother and baby are happy with their nursing relationship, there is no reason to end it right on the baby's first birthday. Many happy nursing pairs nurse well into the second or third year.

## 59 Starting Solids

One of the most exciting milestones in your baby's first year will come when you can begin to give her solid food. The first thing to do is determine when to start feeding solids to your baby. Be sure you don't start too early, as this can cause choking and instigate food allergies. The AAP recommends that you don't start solids until at least six months of age. However, there's not a definite start date; your baby will show signs of readiness, such as interest in food, ability to grab small food pieces between thumb and forefinger, and ability to take food into the mouth without tongue thrusting. These signs usually appear in combination around the sixth month, but don't be fooled by a random early sign.

Once you have decided to start feeding solids to your baby, you'll need to choose which solids to feed. The general consensus is that a low-allergen item like rice cereal is a good starter food. You simply reconstitute the dried cereal with breast milk, formula, or water. Your pediatrician may recommend that you try a couple of other cereals, too, before moving on. After cereals, babies generally move on to vegetables.

After vegetables, you can move on to fruits, and eventually meats, if you wish. Remember to keep each new food separate from others so you can watch for allergies. Of course, be sure textures are not too sharp or hard and serving size pieces are small enough to chew thoroughly and swallow.

## Feeding Your Baby from the Table 60

Now that you've figured out what your baby tolerates and enjoys in terms of food, you can get a bit more creative. Make baby food from scratch and have your baby eat at the table with you and your partner. Making baby food is fun and cost effective, and feeding the baby from the table makes things easier for you. All you need is something to grind food with. A regular food processor will do the trick, but there are also special baby-food grinders on the market.

When you make dinner for the family, simply throw some of the dinner into the baby-food grinder and serve it to your baby. This makes it easier for the baby to swallow and digest the food. Even if your baby has not shown signs of food allergies, discuss with your pediatrician about foods your baby should continue to avoid until she's older. If your baby really likes a dish, consider saving the leftovers.

Eventually you won't need to grind foods for your baby; you will simply be able to feed him from the family's dish of food. As your baby develops teeth and chewing motions (with or without teeth), he will come to enjoy the texture of foods.

**61.** When Your Baby Is Newborn • 80
**62.** The First Month • 81
**63.** Months 2 and 3 • 82–83
**64.** Months 4 and 5 • 84–85
**65.** Months 6 and 7 • 86–87
**66.** Months 8 and 9 • 88–89
**67.** Months 10 through 12 • 90–91
**68.** Offer Tactile Stimulation • 92
**69.** Choose the Right Toys • 93
**70.** Encourage Pretend Play • 94
**71.** Encourage Creativity • 95
**72.** Remember Tummy Time • 96
**73.** What Is Cruising? • 97
**74.** Is There a Problem? • 98
**75.** Seek Help • 99

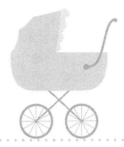

# Part 5

## Physical and Mental Development

One of the best experiences you'll have as a mother is watching your new baby grow. As your baby grows, she will also gain new skills. Many babies reach certain milestones around the same age, while some jump ahead or fall behind the norm. The most important thing to remember is that all babies are different. Crawling, walking, or talking sooner does not necessarily indicate greater intelligence, athleticism, or health than doing so later on.

## 61. When Your Baby Is Newborn

Newborn babies are much more complex than they're given credit for. Though their future skills have not yet become evident, much of the groundwork has already been laid for these abilities. For example, your baby has a fully developed body. What she lacks is coordination and control. This is the reason why she might occasionally slap herself in the face with a flailing arm, or knock into your shoulder as she swings her head around.

One thing you can do to encourage physical development in your newborn is give her lots of skin-to-skin contact. Consider letting her lie in only a diaper on your or your partner's chest. Hearing the familiar sound of a heartbeat and feeling the warmth of your body will relax her, and maybe even put her to sleep. To keep your newborn warm, simply place a blanket over the top of you both. This is important, as newborn babies do not yet have good temperature regulation abilities.

# The First Month

The first month is an adjustment for everyone. Your baby is getting used to extra-uterine life. You and your partner are just starting to figure out your new roles as parents. By the end of the first month, life will begin to settle into a manageable routine.

**Physical Development**

At this point, your baby still does not have much control over his body. You still need to support him as you hold him, particularly his head. His neck muscles are weak, so even when resting on your shoulder, his head can flop around, which can cause damage. Be sure to always hold your baby's head secure. Tummy time will help him learn to develop his neck muscles. Though your baby cannot yet reach for objects, you may notice him staring intently at certain things.

**Mental Development**

Your baby will particularly enjoy looking at faces in this first month. Smiling at your baby may inspire a partial smile in response, though a full smile is not to be expected right away. High-contrast patterns will also amuse a one-month-old.

In terms of voice development, your baby will begin some spontaneous cooing in the first month. At this age, your baby will also cry if over- or understimulated.

## Months 2 and 3

By the second and third months, the postpartum period as most people think of it is coming to an end. Life has found a rhythm and is calming down. However, this doesn't mean that your baby stops changing. Change is constant in a new baby's life.

### Physical Development

Your baby's movements will begin to take on a purpose. Her muscles will begin to relax and her hands uncurl. First, your baby will begin to extend her arms and legs. Then, she will more deliberately extend and retract her limbs. Your baby will also begin to gain control of her head and neck. Your baby may be able to lift her head at about a 45-degree angle.

Your baby may even be able to hold a small object like a rattle for a brief while. This duration will increase in length as time goes on. By the end of the third month, your baby may be rolling one or both ways. So never leave your baby on the couch or any other raised surface.

### Mental Development

Your baby still loves to look at you, and now you are rewarded with intentional coos and giggles. You may notice that your baby's babbling is also taking on a more verbal quality. Listen for some long vowel sounds coming from your baby.

Your baby's personality will also begin to show in the second and third months of life. Your baby will be able to convey basic emotions with facial expression. She will also begin learning cause and effect and making use of that knowledge. For instance, she will learn that if she cries, you will respond. This may become tiring for you, but your baby gets her sense of security from your quick and consistent response.

Crying is not always a bad thing. In fact, crying is an important form of communication. By this point, you will probably have learned that your baby has different cries for different situations: She may cry out when she's hungry, whine and whimper when she's sleepy, and shout to get your attention.

## 64 Months 4 and 5

This is a very exciting age for your baby. He will notice everything in his environment and respond to each thing with great enthusiasm. This is one of the last periods of time where your baby is still largely dependent on you to get around. But watch out, because mobility is close at hand!

### Physical Development

Your baby has much better head and neck control now. Your baby's head really needs support only when he is tired or asleep. Your baby should be able to hold his or her head up to about a 90-degree angle.

Your baby will also begin to move objects from hand to hand. This passing game can last for lengthy periods of time and helps develop hand coordination. Also, with a bit of help your baby can stand up. He will likely roll a lot as well. Eventually, toward the end of this time, your baby may begin to wiggle forward (or backward) on the floor. This is the beginning stage of crawling.

### Mental Development

Your baby is now aware that everything has a name. You may even hear some forms of words coming out of his mouth. When Daddy comes into the room, you may hear your baby say, "Da-da." Don't be sad if it's Dad's name that he calls first. This is normal.

Babies of this age love colors and contact and are captivated by speech. Your baby will laugh hard when tickled or when he finds something funny. Your baby has also developed the ability to communicate his dislikes, usually by pushing away something or making a signal like he's wiping his nose. On the other hand, your baby will also make motions to indicate that he wants to be picked up or played with.

## 65 Months 6 and 7

Watch out world . . . here she comes! During these months your baby will be exploring her mobility options, and reaching for and grabbing things more easily than before. Just make sure you have the house baby-proofed before you let her wander at will.

### Physical Development

Sitting is a skill your baby has been working on and will likely successfully complete during these months. He'll also be able to support himself on his hands and knees. Your baby will be able to reach up and actually get what he is going after as well, which may worry you. Increased fine-motor skills and the pincher grasp (baby uses his thumb and forefinger to pick up small items) will follow.

Plastic baby utensils and dishware are great for babies of this age. Choose spill-proof cups for your little one to use. These items help your baby develop self-feeding skills, which will be perfected in the coming months.

### Mental Development

Your baby is now much more vocal than before. You may even hear some two-syllable sounds coming from your once-quiet child. You might even catch your baby having a conversation with a toy or his reflection. This babbling helps your baby express himself.

Your baby is still a great imitator at this age. He loves mimicking your facial expressions. Don't be surprised if your baby gets anxious when spoken to or held by strangers or people he doesn't know well. A preference for his parents is common among babies at this age. Your baby may also begin to respond to his name at this time.

## 66 Months 8 and 9

At this point in your baby's life, she will look more like a toddler than a baby. She will still crave bonding time with you, but exert a bit more independence. You will notice your little one really flirting with mobility now. Get ready, because crawling is just around the corner.

### Physical Development

You'll see definite signs that crawling is on the way. Once your baby is on hands and knees, you may see her rocking back and forth, as if in anticipation of motion. This is a precrawling posture. Eventually your baby will find a way to propel herself forward.

From rolling both ways to sitting supported and then unsupported, the next step is obvious. It's time to move upward. Around this time, your baby will start pulling herself up with the use of stable objects like furniture. Typically, your baby will be so excited by the accomplishment that she will immediately thump back down again.

### Mental Development

Your baby has learned a lot since birth. Now he may understand that toys or objects may be hidden under a blanket or behind your back. You may also enjoy playing nesting games using stackable cups or dolls with your child. These are really intellectually stimulating and help develop spatial relations.

Language ability is also growing by leaps and bounds. This month you may actually begin to hear a first few words, though some babies are fairly quiet at this age. As long as you hear some babbling, your baby is fine.

## 67 Months 10 Through 12

At this age your baby is a toddler. You'll learn why the name toddler is given to a child of this age as you watch your wobbly little one move about. Things will start to get a little more complicated as your toddler gains access to off-limits items and pulls himself up onto furniture.

### Physical Development

Crawling is mastered by this point. A few babies begin walking at this age, but this is rare. Most babies exhibit a behavior known as cruising, in which they pull themselves up to a standing position using furniture and other steady objects for support and then take small steps as they continue holding on.

From crawling to walking, your baby will learn to stabilize himself and move around. This doesn't mean that falls won't happen, so keep an eye on him as he wobbles around. As your baby masters walking, the falls become less frequent and less traumatic.

### Mental Development

At this time, your baby is a social butterfly. She will be smiling and giggling up a storm. Simple games are lots of fun at this age. A big favorite for your baby will probably be peekaboo—a game she could play for hours. This is also a great game for toddlers to play with babies.

By now your baby's language skills are also more developed. Not only is your baby trying to communicate with words, which you may or may not understand, but your baby is able to understand words. If you point at an object and say the name, your baby is likely to mimic.

One of the words your baby will quickly learn and love to overuse is *no*. Whenever you issue a command, her response will probably be "No." Even if you were to ask, "Would you like a cookie?" "No" is what you'd hear. Don't worry—this defiance lasts only a little while, until she becomes equally infatuated with the word *yes*.

## 68  Offer Tactile Stimulation

Tactile stimulation, or appealing to the baby's sense of touch, is a great thing for even a small child. You don't have to spend lots of money on fancy toys—you can make your own tactile toys. For instance, put a few different objects with different textures into a paper bag. You can choose cotton balls, cereal pieces, one of your baby's socks, or whatever else you have around. Let your baby reach in and hand you an object. Talk to him about the object that he's pulled out. Your baby will love choosing objects and hearing your voice as you explain them.

Tactile foods are also a great idea. As your baby gets older, change the texture of his foods. Watch how he rolls the food around in his mouth and hands. It's a messy process, but it serves to stimulate your baby's brain. Tapioca pudding is one example of a tactile food your baby may love.

## Choose the Right Toys 69

There are very few rules to keep in mind when buying toys for your baby. The main one is that the toys need to be safe. Look out for removable parts that can be swallowed, long strings or cords that can be choking hazards, and other potentially dangerous aspects. The truth is, the simpler the toy, the better it is for a baby. Your little one is more likely to show interest in the box a toy comes in than in the toy itself.

A basic, soft ball is a classic toy for your baby. Even very small babies love to watch a ball roll around. It's great for babies to become acquainted with this common shape early on. An unbreakable mirror is also a great toy. Remember, babies love to look at faces, and they become especially infatuated with their own reflections. Your baby may also start to hold the mirror up to you as he learns what a reflection is. And of course, simple toys that make noise, like bells and rattles, are big favorites. Balls, mirrors, and rattles will all give your baby his first lesson on cause and effect.

It's also nice for baby to have a stuffed animal or doll to play with. However, until your child is out of a crib, he shouldn't take this toy to bed with him. Older babies and toddlers love to play with stuffed toys and dolls and pretend to care for them like pets or children.

## 70 Encourage Pretend Play

Pretend play is so important for your baby. This is one of the best ways for your child to express himself creatively. Your baby will begin pretend play by simple imitation. This begins nearly from birth as your baby begins to imitate facial gestures. From there your baby will begin to learn to move around alone, from rolling to scooting to cruising and finally walking. Each of these physical phases of development will add a new dimension to the pretend play.

To encourage pretend play in your baby, give him plenty of free play. Not every moment of playtime needs to be orchestrated. You can simply set a few small and simple toys down with your baby. Big, fancy toys won't do anything for your baby that simple toys won't. In fact, the more simple a toy is, the more likely your baby is to use his imagination when playing with it.

Babies also love to mimic their parents' daily lives. Popular toys for kids reveal this, as they are often replicas of grownup items like phones, vacuum cleaners, cars, and the like. Encourage this kind of imitation in your child. It means he looks up to you and is interested in your life.

## Encourage Creativity 71

Creativity is the ability of your baby to be expressive in art and music. There are plenty of simple ways to encourage this in your child. The first thing to do is offer your baby creative freedom. Give her a couple of crayons and some blank paper. Coloring books are fun too, but these suggest your child should color within the lines. Blank paper helps children feel free to draw whatever they like.

Musical instruments can make great creative toys as well. Babies can make noise and learn about rhythm. This helps them learn about patterns and mathematics. Eventually, you'll see your little one playing along with the rhythm of a song. Clapping is another variation of this skill development.

## 72 Remember Tummy Time

Tummy time is a way for your child to build muscles in her upper body. As she learns to push up on her arms, she'll gain arm strength. Your baby will also gain strength in her neck muscles, which are used to help your baby lift and turn her head. These are important skills for every baby to learn.

In addition to fundamental development time, tummy time can be playtime—a chance to look around and explore. For very young babies, simply put a mirror to one side and let her enjoy talking to the "other" baby. As your baby gets older and learns to lift her head, other toys may be fun for her. Eventually, as your baby expands her movement base, you can place toys slightly out of her reach so she can practice reaching for the toy.

Don't be afraid to get right down on the floor with your baby. Lie down next to him and talk to him while he's small, or lie head to head and rest on your chin, watching him while he watches you. It is also okay to simply leave the baby to play on his own, as long as you always have him in your sight.

# What Is Cruising? 73

Your baby's physical development can be tracked by her change in movement. Your baby first begins to roll from one side to the other, and then back again. Then your baby learns to sit. Maybe scooting comes next, followed by crawling. The stage between crawling and walking is called cruising. This is where your baby holds on to furniture, people, or whatever she can grab to support herself while she moves around. Each of these milestones is fun and important.

Cruising is a wonderful time of anticipation. It's clear that walking is just around the corner, and you're ready. Perhaps you have cameras poised in every room, waiting to capture those first wild steps and your baby's excited face. However, the cruising milestone is also an important one. Unfortunately, it brings some dangers that you may not be expecting.

Now is when it is very important to get down on your hands and knees and assess your home for potential dangers. Are there glass objects on the table that your baby could grab? What about power cords that could trip the baby or even be chewed on? Can your baby reach the cords hanging from the window blinds?

Anything that could potentially be dangerous to your baby needs to be removed or separated from your baby. This includes gating off areas that could cause problems, like stairs, rooms with slick floors, or rooms with sharp-cornered furniture.

## 74 Is There a Problem?

It's very normal for new mothers to worry that their babies are not developing at a healthy rate. It's also normal to compare your baby to other babies, including siblings and cousins. While all children grow and develop at different rates, certain lapses or deficiencies do indicate that your baby needs to be watched or evaluated more closely by your pediatrician or another health-care provider.

Many times you might think your baby has a problem, but you are unsure. This can really wreak havoc on your life. To be on the safe side, you should seek help as soon as you suspect that there is a problem in your child's development. You might be overly cautious, but it's better to be safe than sorry.

If you think your child might have a problem, do some research. Read books on early child development and compare the information to your child's situation. Discuss your suspicions with friends who have children. If they've noticed similar characteristics in their own children that turned out to be nothing, your child will probably be fine as well.

# Seek Help 75

Where to seek help for your child will depend on what you or your pediatrician thinks is wrong. There are some issues that can be managed within your pediatrician's scope of practice. These may be minor issues common among children of your child's age, such as an innocent heart murmur.

Most major cities have a specialty hospital for children. Here you will find all types of medical specialists who have expertise in anything from disease to developmental issues. Specially trained health-care providers such as physical therapists, occupational therapists, and speech therapists might be able to help with your child's developmental issues. If there isn't a local children's hospital, ask your pediatrician if he knows of any local programs for babies with developmental problems. Many states have specialized agencies just for this purpose. If you have a baby who is at a higher risk of developmental delays because of a preterm birth or other issue, you may be given this information before your baby leaves the hospital.

There are also many national and international organizations for children who have developmental delays or difficulties. These can easily be found online or by asking your practitioner for local resources.

**76.** Avoid Full-Length Mirrors! • 102
**77.** Prepare for Changes in Your Skin • 103–104
**78.** Prepare for Changes in Your Hair • 105
**79.** Your First Period • 106
**80.** Bone Movement • 107
**81.** How to Lose the Baby Weight • 108
**82.** Find Time to Work Out • 109
**83.** Workout Common Sense • 110–111
**84.** Beaware of New Mom Trouble Spots • 112
**85.** Where to Work Out • 113
**86.** Overcome Obstacles • 114
**87.** Fitness Fashion • 115
**88.** Postpartum Plastic Surgery? • 116
**89.** Treat Yourself Right • 117

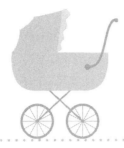

# Part 6

## Post-Baby Body and Fitness

It's happened—the baby is here, and you've finally returned home. After a couple of days of feeling really skinny, you realize that you're only skinny compared to your former nine-month-pregnant self. Now, your belly is saggy where the baby used to live. You have lines and marks all over your body. Your hair is falling out. Your skin is dry. What can you do to look and feel normal again?

## 76 Avoid Full-Length Mirrors!

Part of being kind to yourself these first few months involves taking the time to uncover the beautiful, glowing woman hidden under the wear and tear of pregnancy and birth. This means taking some reasonable precautions. Don't look at yourself naked. Avoid full-length mirrors at all costs. And feel free to wear sweats as often as you like.

Not everyone's body is in terrible shape after birth. How your body looks and feels depends largely on how well you took care of yourself during pregnancy. If you didn't gain excessive weight, you probably won't have much to shed. You may also find you weigh less than prior to pregnancy if you took better care of yourself after becoming pregnant.

Try to focus on where you're going instead of where you have been. Give more attention to the positive aspects of your body. Do you have more curves than you did before your baby was born? Maybe you're enjoying an enhanced bra size? These positives will help you through the tough parts of regaining a healthy and attractive body. The keys to looking good, particularly as a new mom, are creating goals and staying motivated enough to meet those goals through good, healthy habits.

## Prepare for Changes in Your Skin 77

The skin changes in postpartum are usually simply reversals of whatever happened during pregnancy. Most women develop stretch marks, acne, and dry skin during pregnancy, which means big changes to your skin postpartum.

**Stretch Marks**

Stretch marks are basically points in your skin where you were not able to stretch anymore. The indentations of the skin show where your skin gave way to make room for your growing baby. The good news is that the red, raw look of early postpartum stretch marks is not permanent. In fact, most stretch marks fade rather rapidly and become silvery or white.

There are plenty of touted cures for stretch marks, though none of them are very beneficial. Some new procedures have been developed to help you rid yourself of these marks, but pursuing this fix is not always the best idea, particularly if you are considering having more children.

**Acne**

If you started looking like a teenager with serious skin problems while you were pregnant, you'll be glad to know that the acne usually clears up in the first six weeks postpartum. You may find this acne on your face or other oily parts of your body. This is because the hormone levels are returning to normal levels. It will take a bit of time before your skin is completely normal again.

Continue to treat whatever blemishes you have with your own resources. Clean skin is usually the way to go. You may also try some over-the-counter products or a visit to the dermatologist to help stabilize your skin.

**Dry Skin**

Your skin may also feel drier during the postpartum period. This dry skin is also caused by postpartum hormone changes. Treat yourself to a nice bottle of your favorite lotion. As soon as you leave the shower, rub this lotion in, prior to drying off. This can help seal some of the moisture back into your skin.

If you notice skin flaking from your body as well as your face, assess your bath regimen. Are you showering at least every other day? Do you take the time to use a washcloth, loofah pad, or other exfoliating product? These can help remove dead skin cells from your body, allowing the healthy skin beneath to shine through.

## Prepare for Changes in Your Hair 78

During pregnancy, your body was so busy working on the growth of your healthy baby that it neglected to fulfill one of its regular jobs: releasing hair. This means that you might have enjoyed a glorious, full head of hair in pregnancy. The bad news is that all the hair you uncommonly retained during the last nine months is going to go now.

### You're Not Going Bald

While washing your hair in the shower you're probably going to notice clumps of hair coming away in your hand or dotting the floor of the shower. Try not to panic. You are not going bald, even if it looks that way. The hairs that are lost in the immediate postpartum period are the hairs that didn't go during pregnancy. If your hair loss continues at a rapid rate past the first few months postpartum, consider having your thyroid levels checked. In this case, there's a chance your hair loss might not be due to pregnancy at all.

### Treat Yourself

Consider treating yourself to a visit to a nice salon. Spend time talking to a stylist. Tell her what your life is currently like and ask for hair suggestions. She'll probably be able to give you something low maintenance.

## 79 Your First Period

When to expect your period will have a lot to do with how you feed your baby. Breastfeeding mothers tend to have a longer delay in the return of their periods. This is because the hormones of breastfeeding suppress ovulation, which triggers your cycles to begin. Some mothers wait for six months to a year before their periods return. Some nursing mothers find that their periods do not return until their babies go long stretches without nursing, like lengthy periods of sleep at night.

If you are not breastfeeding your baby, you will find that your periods return much sooner. Most nonbreastfeeding mothers will find that they can expect their periods to return about six weeks after the birth.

### Changes to Your Period

Some women do experience changes, with flow and/or cramping. Some of the changes may be for the better though. You may notice that your flow is lighter. You may also experience less cramping than before. The downside is that you could just as easily wind up with more painful periods or a heavier flow. The good news is that problems with your period are usually short-lived and work themselves out within a couple of cycles.

## Bone Movement   80

During the last moments prior to the birth of your baby, you probably felt strong tension in your hip area. This occurred because your hip bones needed to separate to allow your body to give birth to your baby. For this reason, many women notice that their hips seem more prominent after giving birth.

Unfortunately, even if you lose every single ounce of weight you gained in pregnancy, you might never fit into the same clothes. You can even lose extra weight, but to no avail. Don't panic. This doesn't mean your hips are visibly bigger than before. The change is usually fairly imperceptible, except in the tightest of clothes.

### Ribs

What can happen to your hips can happen to your ribs as well. This expansion of your rib cage usually happens toward the end of pregnancy. Rib expansion happens less frequently than hip expansion, but it does happen. The expansion of your ribs is caused by the pressure of your growing uterus in pregnancy. In essence, your ribs move slightly to make room for your baby. You may or may not have experienced sore ribs in pregnancy due to this phenomenon. The good news is that most shirts are forgiving enough that it's rarely noticeable.

# 81. How to Lose the Baby Weight

The combination of a healthy diet and exercise will be your fastest way back to the body you want. There are many different ways for new mothers to work on losing the weight they gained in pregnancy. You may enjoy the group efforts of some diets, such as Weight Watchers, or prefer a stand-alone diet option. No matter what you choose, you can be successful.

### Calories

Burning more calories than you take in is the key to losing weight. Your body burns calories all day; even breathing uses up calories. Find small ways to expend calories during your day, in addition to eating well. Your body is taking on the enormous task of repairing itself. Your body really needs the calories to help repair the damage done by pregnancy, which takes a great toll on your body. During this time, it is very important to eat a balanced diet.

### Breastfeeding Helps

Breastfeeding is one of the best ways to help your body lose weight postpartum. The fat stores that your body accumulated during pregnancy were designed to help you breastfeed. These fat stores won't be tapped into unless you're breastfeeding.

## Find Time to Work Out 82

Don't view working out as a chore. Instead, think of it as a luxury: time spent by yourself working on your own needs and goals. It gives you a chance to get back into that skirt you love, or to reach your ideal mile time. Also, the healthier you are, the more energy you'll have to handle the demands of your new baby. Of course, it won't always be easy. Here are a few tips to guide you through the rough spots.

- Stick to a schedule. Keep a workout appointment with yourself, much as you would keep a dental or hair appointment.
- Incorporate your baby. Take your baby out in the stroller, and speed-walk or jog while pushing the stroller.
- Quick and easy exercise. Take the stairs instead of the elevator whenever you can. Park at the back of the parking lot and walk the rest of the way to the store rather than wait for the perfect spot to open up. Do different exercises during TV commercials.

# 83 Workout Common Sense

Part of the problem with working out after your baby is born is that you probably won't be as protective of your body as you were during pregnancy. Yet, just because the baby has been born does not mean that you can get away with overworking your body at the gym. Remember, you are still recovering from giving birth and must take precautions when getting back into shape.

### Body Changes and Fitness

After a few weeks of recovery, you may feel pumped and ready to get back in the game. You might be excited to pick up where you left off in your running workouts a year ago. It's true that you are able to work out after having a baby. However, you may not be able to exercise as long and as hard as you'd like, due to some body changes.

Relaxin is a pregnancy hormone that helps your body adapt to being pregnant. It allows your joints to be more flexible for ease in giving birth. But once you've had your baby, there is little use for relaxin. The problem is that it takes a while for your relaxin levels to drop. For this reason, you need to take it very easy on your joints; you are more prone to injury during this time.

Be careful that you do not overextend your arms and legs as you work out. If you begin to feel pain during stretching or other activities, stop. This means that you are stretching too far. But don't worry; you should be back to your normal capacity by the three-month mark.

### Common Post-birth Pitfalls

One exercise pitfall that many moms face is not being able to resume their prior physical activity level. You can't simply jump back into the level of exercise you were doing before you got pregnant. Even if you continued to work out throughout your entire pregnancy, you still lost some of your fitness level and muscle mass.

Be sure to ease back into your workouts. Start slowly and gradually increase. Do not attempt to increase the intensity or duration of your physical activities by more than 10 percent per week.

Another common exercise problem for new moms is that they do not eat enough. Because your body will be healing and repairing itself, you will simply need more calories to support increased physical activity. You may be trying to burn calories when working out, but it's very possible to go too far. If you are not adequately nourished, you could suffer from fatigue, dehydration, injury, and other problems.

## 84  Be Aware of New Mom Trouble Spots

Even after you've lost most of the remaining weight from pregnancy, you will probably still have a few weak areas that need attention. For many women, these areas include the abdominal muscles, the hips, and general flexibility in muscles and joints.

### Abdominal Muscles

Your belly is the most obvious area of change in pregnancy. Since this area becomes stretched out during pregnancy, it obviously takes some time and effort to get it back in shape.

Abdominal work can begin within a couple of weeks of birth, assuming that you don't have any separation of the muscles. Start slowly with a few abdominal exercises a day. Slowly increase the amount of repetitions. Once you're comfortable, you can increase the frequency. Luckily, abdominal muscles are very forgiving and can withstand a significant amount of activity.

### Flexibility

There are some very simple exercises you can do in a few spare minutes to regain flexibility in problem areas like your neck, chest, and hips. You can stretch while sitting in front of the computer, watching TV, or folding laundry.

# Where to Work Out

Where you work out is important. Your success in getting in shape depends largely on the space you choose. Factors such as proximity, ease of use, and cost can make or break your plan to get fit. Whether you choose to work out in a gym or a spa, or even in your own home, the important thing is that you create a plan and stick to it.

### Gyms and Spas

Working out at a gym or spa is a fairly popular option. Being surrounded by other people striving to stay healthy can serve as a great source of motivation. You may also find benefits at a local gym or spa, such as specific classes you want to take, workout equipment you may not have at home, and child-care facilities. But gyms may be expensive, so look into various options and compare prices.

### Working Out at Home

Sometimes the best place to work out is right in the privacy of your own home and neighborhood. This option doesn't require a membership fee, but you will have to pay the up-front cost of any equipment you might need. However, you can probably find second-hand equipment for sale in the local paper. The home option allows you to work out on your own schedule, for as long or brief a duration as you like.

## 86 Overcome Obstacles

You may have the determination, the drive, and the physical ability to work out, but other challenges can still stand in your way. If you're lacking time, money, and/or easy child care, your motivation to get in shape may not be enough. Consider the following:

**Time:** If you can't find the time to work out, trick yourself. Allocate a certain number of hours each week to working out and schedule these time blocks on your calendar. Treat these blocks like doctor's appointments and consider them nonnegotiable.

**Money:** You may believe that it takes lots of extra money to work out. The truth is that in most cases, you can work out for only a few dollars a month, or even for free. Use what you already have in the house. Don't buy hand weights; use filled water bottles instead.

**Child care:** If you can't afford a gym with child-care facilities, there are other options to try. Put up a sign in your local grocery store, advertising your desire to pair up with another mom and provide child care while you exercise. With this arrangement, you can work out while she watches your child, and she can work out while you watch hers.

# Fitness Fashion

The clothing you wear while working out will influence your success. Though the easiest and most affordable option is to throw on an old T-shirt and a pair of shorts, well-designed athletic wear can make a big difference. Certain materials keep you comfortable by wicking moisture away from your body. Also, some fabrics allow your skin to breathe while you work out. Not only will you feel better wearing quality clothing, but these items can actually allow you to work out more safely and effectively.

In addition to choosing clothes made of the right materials, you need to make sure they fit well. Clothes that are too tight can restrict your breathing and trap body heat. Clothes that are too big and baggy could cause you to trip and fall, and the extra fabric might make you overheat.

### Shoes

The shoes you wear should correspond with the type of exercise you do. For example, if you do running workouts, you want to ensure that you wear proper running shoes. You need plenty of cushion and support to handle the stress on your feet, ankles, and knees. There are also specific shoes made for walking, tennis, hiking, and aerobics. If you do a variety of sports, consider investing in a pair of cross trainers.

## 88 Postpartum Plastic Surgery?

Plastic surgery may seem like the easy answer to all of your postpartum body-image issues. Even a night in the hospital might not sound too bad at this point. However, most postpartum moms are not great candidates for plastic surgery, at least not right away. If you choose to have surgery, you will have a preliminary meeting with the surgeon to discuss the issues you have and their potential solutions. The surgeon will also take photographs and document your health history.

### The Right Weight

One of the biggest issues will be your weight. The majority of good plastic surgeons will not even consider working with you until you're at or near your ideal body weight because surgery won't really help or last if you aren't close to this weight when you have the procedure. Liposuction and other plastic surgery methods are not meant to help you lose weight. These surgeries are designed to help reshape and contour your body. Being overweight when you have surgery adds risks to your surgery, including the potential of poor wound healing.

## Treat Yourself Right 89

It can be so easy to become totally focused on your baby in those first few months after birth. While loving and caring for your baby is never a bad thing, it is also important to take care of yourself. Don't neglect your own needs during this time.

Some of the biggest complaints from new moms relate to physical stress: the strain of lost sleep, the physical changes to the body, the inability to focus or concentrate. Taking care of yourself can help relieve these issues. Of course, this doesn't mean you should abandon your family each day and spend six hours in a spa. Instead, consider doing small things for yourself to regain balance and control.

For instance, while the baby naps, avoid the laundry and grab a good book to read instead. Consider writing a letter to a friend you've lost touch with. Don't do the dishes. Instead, paint your nails and rub some lotion on your sore legs and shoulders. In short, do what you need to do to stay healthy and in a good mood.

**90.** Love Your Mom Body • 120
**91.** Are You Physically Ready? • 121–122
**92.** Your Six-Week Checkup • 123
**93.** Are You Emotionally Ready? • 124
**94.** Hormone Fluctuations • 125
**95.** The First Time • 126
**96.** Choose Positions that Make You Comfortable • 127–128
**97.** Whining Versus Wining • 129
**98.** Find Time to Be Together • 130
**99.** Rekindle the Romance • 131
**100.** What to Do When You Have a Headache • 132
**101.** How Frequently Should You Have Sex? • 133
**102.** Birth Control: Barrier Methods • 134
**103.** Birth Control: Hormonal Methods • 135–136
**104.** Permanent Birth Control • 137–138
**105.** Breastfeeding as Birth Control • 139

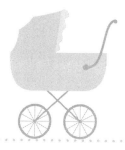

# Part 7

## Sex after Baby

Probably one of the last things on your mind after you have your baby will be sex. You'll have a ton of things requiring your attention, particularly the needs of your newborn baby. You won't be getting much sleep, and your body will still be returning to normal. But don't worry—the feelings of love and affection will return. You and your partner do remember what life was like before the baby came, and postpartum sex will become a reality.

# 90 Love Your Mom Body

When all the weight is gone, all the stretch marks have faded, and all the flab has re-formed into firm skin, your new mom body will be evident. Short of drastic measures like plastic surgery, this is the new you. Do what you can to make loving your mom body an easier transition.

### Makeover

Consider a new mom makeover for yourself. Get a new hairstyle and a new bottle of perfume. Even if you're not a big fan of makeup, just a bit of lip gloss and some eye shadow can make you feel glamorous. You don't even have to spend a fortune on this. Many cities have department stores or independent consultants who will provide you with a free makeover just for learning about their products. Do this with a friend for a fun afternoon activity.

In addition to making over your body, make a change in your overall outlook. Look at your body and your baby with fresh eyes and put any pain from pregnancy and labor behind you. Embrace the new you and move forward with your life. Learning from first pregnancies can help you make changes in future pregnancies.

# Are You Physically Ready?

Most sources you consult will give you a generic six-week rule before you can have sex after birth. Yet, while six weeks may be just the right amount of time for one person, it may be too long or too short for you. When assessing your physical preparedness to resume sex, you must consider several factors. First, you need to consider how you gave birth. Giving birth vaginally may provide you with certain reasons to be cautious about resuming sex. A cesarean birth would provide you with a different reason to be cautious.

### Bleeding

Bleeding or other discharge from your vagina indicates that your uterus is not done healing. If you have any discharge, you should not engage in sexual intercourse. If you're unsure if you've been bleeding for a normal length of time, do not hesitate to call your doctor or midwife.

Once you have quit bleeding or your discharge has stopped, you can usually be cleared to have sexual intercourse. If you see a return to bleeding, you must stop. This may be a return of your normal menstrual cycle if it has been longer than six weeks, or it may be a sign that you were not truly healed.

### Perineum

Obviously, giving birth can cause trauma to your perineum. If you did not have an episiotomy or require a repair, your perineum will heal more quickly and you will have less likelihood of infection. Your perineum should feel normal within a week or two after birth.

If you had an episiotomy or required stitches in the perineum after birth, you may take longer to heal. This can also make you very nervous when you begin to think about having sexual intercourse again. The good news is that even after an episiotomy or repair, your perineum will probably be healed within six weeks of giving birth. Just don't be surprised if you still feel sore for a while, even after you are completely healed.

### Incision

If you gave birth via cesarean surgery, you might feel like you've lucked out of the problems associated with the perineum. That is true. However, you will need to pay attention to your incision. Sexual intercourse can place an extra strain on your incision, even though it's not located around your vagina.

You will want to ensure that your incision is free from redness and that it is not tender prior to even thinking about sex. If your incision is red, tender, or seems to leak or seep fluid, call your doctor. These may be signs of infection.

## Your Six-Week Checkup  92

After nine long months filled with visits to your practitioner's office, you will have one final visit. This will consist mainly of a physical exam. The following are a few procedures and issues that may be performed or discussed at this time:

**Pap smear:** This will give your practitioner a chance to look at your perineum. She can talk to you about how this area is healing, if you required any stitches from an episiotomy. Your practitioner should discuss the resumption of sexual activity as well.

**Breast exam:** During this exam, the practitioner will be looking for irregularities or masses that have appeared since your last exam. You can also ask any breastfeeding questions you may have and inquire about doing breast self-exams while nursing.

**Followup procedures:** If you require any followup lab work or procedures such as hernia repair, now is the time to discuss them with your practitioner. You may also need to have some immunizations; the one new mothers commonly need is the rubella vaccine.

**Birth control:** Bring any questions you have about birth control with you. Consider writing them down so you don't forget.

## 93. Are You Emotionally Ready?

After giving birth, most women feel completely drained of energy. After giving of yourself all day to a tiny human being who requires so much care, the last thought on your mind in the evening is cuddling up with your partner. The good news is that this feeling doesn't last forever.

In fact, talking to your partner about your predicament can actually help solve the problem. Maybe he can offer to bathe the baby after dinner and play with him a bit so you can enjoy a luxurious shower alone. Maybe even a nice walk alone or trip to the store would be helpful in refreshing your spirit. You may find that once you get a bit of time to yourself, you will feel like a completely different person. A few minutes each evening can be enough for you to recharge and find that you really do have some extra energy to spend with your partner, whether or not that means sex.

Talking about your feelings—and his—is a very important part of preparing for your new sexual relationship. If you each understand how the other is feeling, then it becomes easier to deal with these personal issues. This will also help ensure that when you do resume intercourse, you both feel comfortable with the situation.

## Hormone Fluctuations 94

It is said that patience is a virtue, and this holds true for the postpartum period. There isn't much you can do about hormone fluctuations except hang on for the ride. However, there are a few handy tips that can help you deal with the mood swings and physical exhaustion.

Primarily, it is very important that you eat well. No matter how busy you get, never skip meals. Eat a variety of healthy, natural foods and be sure you are getting the recommended daily supply of vitamins and minerals. This will help your body heal and make you feel better.

Another tip is to sleep whenever you can. You may not get a full night's sleep very often, but even several bursts of a few hours each day can work for you. Getting sufficient sleep helps your body heal and keeps you in a rational frame of mind.

For most new mothers, the hardest part is the first few days. If you can manage to laugh at some of the ridiculous things you think and feel during those first few days, the rest will be a breeze.

## 95 The First Time

You and your partner have decided that you are both physically and emotionally ready to have sexual intercourse again. In some ways, it's like being a virgin all over again. You're both nervous. You've got to find the right time and the right place. Your partner is probably worried about hurting you, and you might be worried about getting pregnant again.

Finding the right time to have sex can be difficult. Do you wait until you're both exhausted at the end of the day simply because the baby will be asleep? Or do you wait for a weekend when Grandma can come take the baby for a long walk? There are no easy answers to this dilemma. You and your partner need to figure out what works best for you. Again, keeping an open line of communication is key to a positive experience.

If the baby is in the house when you have sex, it is quite possible that in the middle of it all, your baby will wake up crying and screaming. In this case, you'll need to decide whether to finish quickly or to satisfy the baby and quickly return to bed. This choice is a tough one, and you may have several unsuccessful sexual encounters before it finally goes according to plan.

## Choose Positions that Make You Comfortable

Prior to the birth of your baby, you may have had some favorite positions. There is no reason to throw these out the window after having a baby. In fact, there are no off-limits positions in the postpartum period. The only exception is lack of comfort.

If you are worried about pain from actual penetration, you may decide to choose a woman-on-top position or a side-lying position. Both of these positions allow for a more shallow penetration. If you decide to be on top, you will have more control over how deep penetration goes and how quickly penetration happens.

If you had a cesarean, you may wish to use a woman-on-top position to prevent pressure from being placed on your incision. This may be more comfortable for you and your partner for a while, but in time you'll be able to use other positions just as comfortably.

Sometimes your breasts may leak as you have an orgasm. This is perfectly normal. You can choose to wear a bra with pads for the first couple of encounters or you can elect to keep a blanket or towel nearby in case you need it. An alternative would be to assume a rear-entry position, perhaps on your hands and knees. If your partner is behind you, he cannot see the milk leaking and you can simply let it fall onto a towel.

# 96

If any position you try is painful, reassess the situation. Do you need to add a bit of personal lubricant? Lubricating the vagina can make penetration easier and less painful. Of course, the best personal lubricant is natural. This type of lubricant is released during orgasm. This being the case, you might try ensuring that you have an orgasm before attempting penetration.

Whatever you do, make sure to keep your sense of humor during the first few encounters after birth. From leaking breasts and crying babies to a large helping of personal lubricant, postpartum sex is definitely a bit different from your usual experience. The good news is that it does eventually work itself out.

## Whining Versus Wining 97

Sometimes your partner might decide that he can whine about not having sex as often as he would like it. This can be very difficult on your relationship. In fact, it may even make you less inclined to have sex with him. Here's an old trick: Rather than whining, remind him about wining and dining. Ask him to put a bit of romance into your lives. Whether it's flowers, poetry, or a clean bathtub, he should do it.

Once you communicate openly on the subject, you'll probably experience a lot more wining than whining. The foundation of many problems between a partner and wife is a lack of communication. The two of you experience your baby's birth and early life very differently, so it makes sense that you would not be on the same page.

## 98 Find Time to Be Together

Adding a new little one to your life can seem to take over every available moment. The truth is, where there's a will, there's a way. As your baby gets older, she will begin to sleep for longer stretches of time. Figure out when you can anticipate these stretches and plan accordingly. You can also consider asking for reinforcements. If your parents or siblings are dying for a chance to take your child out for a walk, give it to them.

However, there is also something to be said for spontaneity. While the above methods will get you through in a pinch, you have to remember that your life will not always involve planning when and where to have sex. This is a temporary solution. Sometimes the mood will strike and the timing will be off. Be wild. Take chances. Occasionally it will all work out perfectly. Occasionally you'll both wind up a bit frustrated or laughing about how everything turned out. No matter what, there is never any harm in trying!

## Rekindle the Romance  99

The key to keeping the flames burning is keeping romance alive. Now that you have your attention more divided because you're a mom, you're going to have to adapt. Don't panic, moms are good at adapting. You're going to be no different.

Try to remember to spend five minutes a day being romantic with your partner. This can be something as simple as a full-bodied kiss goodbye in the morning as opposed to the half-focused peck on the cheek. You'd be surprised what a bit of body contact will do. Also, consider slipping a love note into his lunch or brief case. If you can't find any paper or you're too embarrassed to send a note in crayon, consider sending a love note via e-mail.

When you're having dinner, try playing footsie. Bring some candles to the table one night, even if you're serving leftover takeout food. Or serve dinner after the baby is in bed and play nice music. Dancing in your pajamas doesn't have to be unromantic; this may rekindle some spark between you. Once your partner sees the effort you are making, it will be much easier for him to put the right foot forward. Don't be surprised if he starts planning surprises of his own.

## 100 What to Do When You Have a Headache

Surely, you're familiar with the headache excuse. The fact is that sometimes you just don't want to have sex. This happened before your baby was born and it will happen afterward. Your new role as a mom isn't necessarily at fault for your lack of sexual desire. Sometimes you and your partner are just on different wavelengths in this department.

Talking to your partner about the fact that you don't always have matching libidos and that it may not be because of the baby is imperative. He may believe that the baby is taking his place in your life. He won't know this isn't the case unless you tell him.

It may take a while for you and your partner to get back on track. In the meantime, consider alternatives to sex. Sometimes snuggling is a nice happy medium. You may find that this meets his need for physical companionship and meets your need for affection without actual intercourse.

However, cuddling may not always do the trick. If he is really in the mood for sex and you are not, there are still alternatives. You can consider sending him off to take a cold shower. Or you could offer to shower with him and give him a chance to take care of his needs through masturbation. Remember to be considerate and respectful of his needs, just as you'd like him to be toward yours.

## How Frequently Should You Have Sex? 101

One thing most people seem to disagree on is how often a couple should have sex. Some people might feel that once every two weeks is sufficient, while others might argue that every other day is more like it. The truth is that there isn't one right amount of sexual contact to have. What works for you and your partner is the perfect amount. It really is the old argument of quality versus quantity.

If you and your partner are okay with the amount of sex you're having, why listen to what others feel is right? This goes even for national studies. If you're having less sex but enjoying it more, who cares? Do only what's best for you and your partner.

Sometimes you may find that your sex life is improved after having a baby. This could be because giving birth has changed your body and made it more pleasurable to have sex or easier for you to achieve an orgasm. It could also be because you know your body better now that you've had a baby. Either way, enjoy it!

## 102 Birth Control: Barrier Methods

Barrier methods of birth control are very common. They are easy to obtain and relatively inexpensive. Most methods require at least some thought prior to having sex, though spontaneity is not completely out the window.

### Condoms

Condoms protect you from pregnancy by preventing the sperm from reaching the egg. They are about 88 percent effective in preventing pregnancy. If you decide to use a condom with spermicide, you can further decrease chances of pregnancy.

Condoms can be kept around your house and used with water-based personal lubricants. You will need to have them handy for when you want to have sex. This is also a great way to make sex a bit less messy.

# Birth Control: Hormonal Methods

The hormonal methods of birth control are all prescriptive items. There are many new ones out today, each with a different hormonal combination. Only your doctor or midwife can help you find the right combination for you.

### Oral Contraceptives (The Pill)

The pill is considered to be about 97 percent effective in preventing pregnancy when taken correctly. There are multiple formulas available for use today. This method of birth control allows for spontaneous sex, but requires that you remember to take a pill at the same time every day. Every missed or late pill can increase your chances of getting pregnant.

There are other considerations to take into account when thinking about the pill. One would be that while you are nursing, you might wish to consider using progesterone-only (mini) pills. Some forms of oral contraceptives can decrease your milk supply. Be sure to let your doctor or midwife know that you are nursing.

### Intrauterine Device (IUD)

The intrauterine device is a piece of shaped metal wire. Your midwife or doctor places the IUD into your uterus during a vaginal exam. The IUD prevents pregnancy by discouraging implantation into the uterine lining. Some IUDs actually release hormones as well.

### Patches, Rings, and Things

Other delivery systems for hormones are via the patch or a ring. These are both prescriptive medications provided by your practitioner. However, they do not require any action before you have sex. They are always in place.

The patch is simply worn on your hip or shoulder. It delivers a continuous amount of medication through your skin. The patch is changed once a week. It is barely noticeable on the skin and is not worn in an obvious area.

A ring is actually inside the vagina. It also delivers hormones to prevent ovulation. Both of these methods of birth control are easier to use than traditional oral contraceptives.

You may also opt for injectable hormones. They can be given monthly or every three months, depending on your prescription. This requires a visit to your practitioner.

# Permanent Birth Control

Since permanent birth control is considered just that, permanent, you should be very sure you are done having children before opting to have this procedure. Many couples wait until their youngest child is at least a year old before making that decision. Others are completely fine with having permanent birth control done during the birth or shortly afterward. Most forms cannot be undone with much success, despite attempts at reversal surgeries for both men and women.

### Vasectomy

Vasectomy is permanent surgical sterilization for a male. This procedure involves altering the vas deferens on each side of your partner's scrotum and interrupting the flow of sperm to the penis. This is usually done very quickly and easily in a urologist's office. It is considered 99 percent effective in preventing pregnancy.

Many men can have this done on Friday and return to work easily on Monday. Ice packs and tight pants (to prevent bouncing) can be very helpful for dealing with discomfort. Talk to a urologist for more information.

## 104

**Tubal Ligation**

This is female surgical sterilization. It is considered to be more than 99 percent effective in preventing pregnancy. Female sterilization is more complicated surgery than male sterilization.

This surgery involves interrupting the pathway of the egg to the uterus. It can be done after a vaginal birth, while you are still in the hospital, though it will increase your recovery time. You may be a candidate for what is called "Band-Aid" surgery, or laproscopic surgery, which consists of small incisions in three or four locations on your abdomen. If you are not a candidate for this type of surgery, it will be required that you have a more open procedure, much like the surgical incision for a cesarean section. You can also choose to have this done after the postpartum period.

## Breastfeeding as Birth Control

Breastfeeding can be used as a method of birth control. This method takes a lot of research on your part before it can be effective. By using the signs of your body and fertility awareness, you can accurately predict when you will begin ovulation.

The basics of using breastfeeding as birth control are not hard to follow, but there are quite a few rules. Your baby cannot have supplemental feedings by bottle, no matter what the bottle contains. He also cannot use a pacifier. Additionally, your baby must have free access to the breast, particularly at night. By letting your baby regulate when he nurses, your body responds by suppressing ovulation. Be sure to read up on this method for other very important rules that must be followed to prevent pregnancy.

**106.** Ease Back into Work • 142
**107.** Pumping at Work • 143
**108.** Consider an Alternative Schedule • 144
**109.** Maintain a Balance • 145
**110.** How to Handle Your Separation Anxiety • 146
**111.** How to Handle Your Baby's Separation Anxiety • 147
**112.** Wish You Were Home? • 148
**113.** Make the Most of Your Time Together • 149
**114.** Choose Child Care Carefully • 150–151
**115.** Learn About Day Care • 152–153
**116.** Family as Child Care • 154
**117.** Consider an Au Pair • 155
**118.** All about Nannies • 156
**119.** Hiring Babysitters • 157
**120.** Monetary Issues with Child Care • 158–159

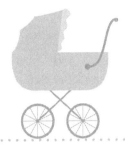

# Part 8

## Working and Child Care

Returning to work as a new mother can be both a blessing and a curse. There are many reasons why you might be going back to work, from finances to the simple fact that you want to work. Even if work is where you want to be, it can be a difficult transition for even an experienced mother. In most cases, families also have to consider the issue of child care if one or both parents work outside the home.

## 106 Ease Back into Work

During pregnancy, you must to talk to your supervisor or Human Resources Department at work about your maternity-leave plans. They may not require anything written in stone. Sometimes they simply ask for an estimate of the time you anticipate taking off, knowing that once your baby is born, things may change. Once your baby has arrived, have a plan in place to let people at work in on the good news. This also allows them to plan to cover your duties during your maternity leave.

Also, you should have a way to stay in touch during your maternity leave so that you can update your employer as needed. This should not, however, be a time to catch up on work. You might consider e-mailing your boss every week or couple of weeks, however, to say, "Hey, I'm still alive, and here's the plan."

When you are within a week or two until your return, talk to your employer about setting a date to come back. Starting back to work toward the end of the week can help ease your transition back to work. Consider working a half day on Thursday and a full day on Friday. This gives you an easy week with enough time to work out issues at home. It also gives you a very nice break on the weekend.

## Pumping at Work 107

Using a breast pump at work shouldn't be scary or worrisome. There are many ways to pump discreetly and easily while at work. If you have your own office, you can simply shut your door. If you have a lock, use it if you think someone might enter. Some mothers hang a sign on the door saying simply "Do Not Disturb"; others hang signs that proudly declare "Pumping in Progress." Your sign can be as bold or as mild as you need it to be to ensure your privacy.

If you do not have your own office, you will need to find a space that works for you. Some businesses actually provide rooms for pumping moms. Check with your employer to see if you can help set one up in your workplace.

If there's no pumping room available, perhaps there's a vacant office or meeting room you can use for short periods of time. Check for any available space. Also, be sure to get clearance from your supervisor to do this; you don't want a group of coworkers banging down the door for a meeting while you're holed up inside pumping. Another alternative would be to pump at the day care or other place your child is during the day. Sometimes you may even be able to get a true feeding in, if your work location is close to your baby's.

# 108 Consider an Alternative Schedule.

With today's technologies, it is very easy to stay connected to your office. Nearly every home has not only a phone but also a computer with some form of Internet connection. If you are able to connect to the Internet from home, it may be quite possible for you to effectively work from home some of the time.

Having a home office is not necessarily easy. It does take some work to figure everything out. Sometimes you may find that work calls you, even though you'd rather be with your family. Having twenty-four-hour access to work can have that effect. Setting "office hours" even when you're home can help alleviate this distraction.

### Job Sharing

Sharing your job with someone else might also be another option for flexibility at work. Perhaps you each work two full days and split the last day each week. Some jobs have you alternate three- and two-day weeks. Another schedule that might work for you would be five half days. Be creative. Find a way to work out your schedule. Be sure that you are capable of getting all the work done. Talk to your supervisor about your idea. She may have someone else in the office who is already willing to do part-time/job-sharing work, or she may be willing to find someone to share your job with you.

## Maintain a Balance

The hard part about working is that you're not done when you come home. Unfortunately, your job as a mother is not nine to five—it continues around the clock. There's no way you can handle all your responsibilities without help. Your primary partner in child care is your partner, so the two of you should divide up the work that needs to be done.

### Sharing the Workload

One of the hardest parts of having a baby, whether you work outside of the home or not, is the division of labor within your home. No matter if one or both parents work, there are still chores to be done at home. Meals have to be made, laundry must be washed, home repairs must be taken care of, and bills must be paid. Who will do what?

Find any way that works for the both of you and divide the chores. Think of everything that needs to be done to run your household. Make a list and check it twice. You may wish to trade some chores back and forth. This works particularly well for the chores that no one wants. Once you have done this, your house will run much more smoothly. You and your partner can quit fighting about dishes and get back to real life.

## 110 How to Handle Your Separation Anxiety

Whether you want to be at work or you have to be at work, you are there. The separation from your baby can be worse if you'd rather not be at work, but either way, you may still miss your baby. There are several things you can do to help ease the pain of separation.

For one, bring a picture or two of your baby to work. Place these where you might normally see them, like your desk or your locker. You might even consider wearing a locket with your baby's picture tucked safely inside. The frequent sight of your baby's face will help you transition into days of separation.

A must for getting used to being away from your baby is having absolute confidence in your child care. A little nervousness is natural, but if you are sincerely worried about your baby's well-being while you're at work, you're not going to get much work done.

Also consider visiting your child or having your partner visit your child during the day.

The truth is that many moms have trouble dealing with initial separation from their babies. It usually gets easier with time, but if you feel that you are not getting any more comfortable with the situation, get help. If you have continually intrusive thoughts about your baby during the day, to the point of not being able to work or concentrate, consider talking to your doctor or midwife.

## How to Handle Your Baby's Separation Anxiety

Most babies are blissfully unaware that their parents have gone to work during the day. They are aware of their new surroundings and the new people around them, but it is usually not distressing to them. What may be distressing to your baby is a change in the lifestyle they were used to having.

Did you pick a child-care facility that will listen to what your baby's schedule has been? Do they have enough people or few enough babies to give your baby the attention he needs? As long as your very young baby has his needs met, he should not become stressed over being someplace other than with you. However, as your baby gets older, separation anxiety can become a very real issue. This can happen as early as about six months. It can also happen later, or your baby may skip it all together.

# 112. Wish You Were Home?

Perhaps you've always been the working type, but now that you've had a baby, you've changed your mind. Maybe you've always wanted to stay home, but you didn't feel like your circumstances would allow it. Either way, you may want to be home right now.

### Making Your Way Home

You may not have even realized that you wanted to be home until after you had your baby and went back to work. This is rather common among new mothers.

Once you know that you'd like to stay home with the baby, discuss this with your partner. Perhaps the two of you can come up with a workable solution. Then take action as soon as you can.

### Dealing with Disappointment

Sadly, no matter how hard you look, there may not be a way for you to stay home. This can be very disappointing, especially if you've gotten your hopes up.

One way to provide some light at the end of the tunnel is to plan for the future. Just because your financial or home situation isn't compatible with your staying home right now, that doesn't mean it won't ever be. Just keep your eyes open for future opportunities to try your plan again.

## Make the Most of Your Time Together

When both you and your partner work, chores are not the only thing that may need to be divided. Sometimes you may find that you are both fighting over time with your baby. This can be an awkward situation. You are both the baby's parents, and your little one needs both of you.

### Dads Matter

Part of the problem with working full-time is that by the end of the day, there may be relatively few hours left when your baby is awake. By the time you've sat down and had dinner, it will probably be time for your baby to go to bed. As a mother, you have the advantage of nonnegotiable nursing time with your baby. Dads, on the other hand, have a trickier situation.

You may be tempted to leave your partner chores disguised as bonding time with the baby. Yet, bathing and diapering are not ideal times to connect with your baby. Your partner needs time to read to, cuddle with, and play with your baby just as much as you do. Try to work out a plan that gives you both the bonding time you need with your baby.

# 114 Choose Child Care Carefully

There are more decisions to make today than ever before when it comes to child care. With all of the options available to you, you may feel like you're swimming in choices. This doesn't necessarily make your decision any easier. In fact, it may seem to complicate things for you. However, there are ways to help yourself in this regard.

**Know Your Options**

Before you make a decision, you need to fully explore all of your options. Look at what is available around you. Do not limit yourself to only what you see on the surface. Are there professional organizations in your area? Home day cares? Leave no stone unturned while searching for the best option for your family.

Ask people you know what types of child-care options they know of in your area. Talk to the people who you work with and those who your partner works with. Talk to the childbirth educators in your area, as they often work with new families and may be aware of other options.

You may think of looking for child care near your home. That is never a bad option, but it can limit you. Do not forget to look at choices for child care near your workplace or your partner's workplace.

You may also find a perfectly good location at the halfway mark, so do not limit yourself too much geographically.

### Questions to Ask

One of the best ways to gather information is to ask questions. First, you need to question yourself: What types of care do you know about? Which do you think matches your child? How would you explain your theories on child-rearing to a child-care provider? What hours do you need? Are you flexible?

Once you've gotten the basics down of what you need for your baby and family, it is time to start figuring out which type of care is right for you. Do you prefer that your baby be in your home? Someone else's home? A day care? Do you want your child alone or with other children? What policies does the facility have for sick children and sick care providers? What are the hours of the facility? Or how many hours can a single provider work per week? What about feeding your baby? How much will it cost?

## 115 Learn about Day Care

The licensed facility that houses numerous children, usually broken down into groups by age, is probably one of the most well-known types of child care. There are some chains that are nationally known and others that are local. Your state or local authorities should license all of these facilities. Be sure to ask to see copies of their current licenses if they are not posted.

### The Benefits

Day care offers many benefits, though some will vary depending on the facility you choose. One of the biggest benefits is that someone will always be there, even if a certain worker is ill or needs vacation time. This can be a very big issue for you, depending on the flexibility you have at your job.

You may also enjoy the routine that has proven effective through use for a long period of time. If this is a national chain, you know that there was probably a lot of thought put into the curriculum, even for the infant ages. This curriculum probably follows a pattern throughout the year.

Another nice thing about a day-care setting is the other children. Even in the youngest age group, your baby is likely to have others around of the same age. Many of these children will stay together as they grow, providing long-term relationships for your baby.

### The Drawbacks

Yes, there is a downside to day care as well. One drawback many parents talk about is the inflexibility of the schedules. If your day care closes before you leave work and your job doesn't have rigid quitting times and there are days you need to stay late, this can cause a problem. You may also have a job where you work certain holidays but the day care is closed.

If your child is sick, you cannot bring her to day care. In fact, most facilities have a twenty-four-hour rule. This means that if your child was sent home sick in the morning on Tuesday, your child can't come back to day care for twenty-four hours after the last symptoms disappeared, which may mean more than one missed day of work.

One of the biggest drawbacks to day-care facilities is the mass-market feel. Your child may get less individualized care and attention than she may get in other child-care settings.

## 116  Family as Child Care

The opportunity to use your family as child care may present itself while you are pregnant. Your loving mother or mother-in-law might begin to drop delightful hints about how wonderful it would be to watch the baby while you go to work. For many families, this works out very well.

You typically pay your family members less (if at all) to help out while you work. They are also usually more flexible in terms of hours. Your baby will be either in your home or in another home that is familiar to him.

This option usually results in fewer sick days, due to your baby's lack of exposure to other children. However, if the family member you have chosen is sick one day, you are left high and dry. Obviously, planned away dates can be worked around, but it's often these unexpected days off that can be troublesome.

There are also bigger problems with using your family for child care. One of the toughest problems can be if your philosophies in child-rearing don't match. It's much harder to have control over a family member than over other providers.

Another real problem with family members as child-care providers occurs when they do not work out. Part of this is because it is personal. Termination of such a child-care situation can be awkward and hurtful for one or both parties.

## Consider an Au Pair 117

Au pairs usually come from au pair agencies located around the world. The amount of training and experience of each au pair may vary wildly, as will the language your au pair speaks, depending both on the agency and the au pair.

### A Stranger in Your House

Having someone live with you can be a blessing. You never have to worry about your au pair being on time for work. Your au pair can play with your baby in familiar surroundings. And your au pair is with your baby and family a lot, so you know what kind of person he is.

While having your au pair around can be very handy for last-minute trips, it can also be a bad situation. Remember, most au pairs are allowed to work for only about forty-five hours per week. It is easy to overwork your au pair by accident, and this will put you in violation of contract.

Having a stranger in your house can be hard to adjust to. Not only will you lose some privacy, but you will also have to put up with this person's personal lifestyle and habits. You may not approve of her choice of music or friends. Be absolutely sure about this person before entering into a contract.

## All about Nannies

The concept of a nanny may seem outdated to you, but this is actually still a popular option. You may opt for a live-in nanny or a nanny who comes in daily to help you out.

### The Benefits

One of the biggest benefits of a nanny is that your child receives one-on-one care from the same person every day. This can be a huge advantage for some families. This is particularly true if you have special requests or your child has special needs.

A nanny may also provide you with extra services. Obviously, you need to preplan these with your nanny, but you might ask for such services as laundry, light (or not so light) housecleaning, dishes, errands, and others. What you pay your nanny should be commensurate with her duties.

### Nanny Training

There are actually nanny schools popping up in several areas around the country. These schools teach things like the basics of child development, infant and child CPR and first aid, infant care, and other important skills.

Other nannies have simply gotten on-the-job training. Decide which type of nanny is right for you.

# Hiring Babysitters

Even if you do not need regular child care, babysitters are common for nearly every parent. Consider your options.

### The Neighborhood Teen

Often a local teen girl in the neighborhood is adequate for most families when it comes to babysitting needs. The local babysitter's training is likely on-the-job experience in conjunction with the caretaking of younger siblings. Yet, some communities do offer Red Cross babysitting training. This training teaches teens about the basics of child care, safety, and even some marketing skills.

### Babysitting Services

The nice thing about babysitting services is that they do all the screening for you. They also hunt down someone for whatever dates and times you may need.

You will usually pay a bit more for the service than you might pay your neighborhood teens. There are also usually a minimum number of hours that they will work, so if you don't stay out that long, you still have to pay for it. Sitters from a service are usually older and have more experience, but the drawback is that you might not have a chance to meet them until they show up at your door, ready to work.

## 120 Monetary Issues with Child Care

There is no doubt about it: Child care costs money. You will be paying for a valuable service, and this service can come at quite a high price. Trying to figure out how much to budget for child care can be a difficult task. This is particularly true if you don't have a real clue about current child-care costs. Begin researching different child-care costs for day care, au pairs, nannies, or babysitters as soon as you become pregnant. Consider the following information about the costs of each option:

**Day care:** Day-care costs will depend on whether it is a chain or a large day care versus a family-run day care. You may also receive cost breaks as your child grows. Some chains even run coupons or offer price breaks for referrals to other parents.

**Family care:** Family care can be free or low cost. Just remember that you might get exactly what you pay for. Even if a family member begs to babysit for free, you might consider insisting on a pay rate to keep the arrangement professional.

**Au pairs:** The weekly cost of an au pair is not as much as other child care, but there are hidden costs. There is the agency fee and the fee for health insurance for the au pair, not to mention basic room and board.

**Nannies:** Nannies may cost the same or a bit less than day care. The good news is that the price may be the same for one child as for two or three. There is also less likelihood that the nanny will charge based on the age of the child.

One of the benefits of having to pay for child care is that there are certain tax incentives available. What type of tax incentive and how much of an incentive it really is will depend on many factors. Part of this is based on the cost of child care, your annual combined income, and other factors.

The Flexible Spending Account (FSA) is a great way to save money on child care. You choose the amount you wish to set aside for child care by taking a pretax portion out of each paycheck. You then apply to receive these funds back over the course of the year.

However, once you have placed the money aside, it is difficult to change your elections for deductions during the year. You usually have to wait for open enrollment to make changes. You will also be unable to get a regular tax break on monies that have been reimbursed through your FSA.

**121.** The Decision to Stay Home • 162
**122.** If It's Not Your Choice • 163
**123.** Should Dad Stay Home? • 164
**124.** Take a Look at Your Finances • 165
**125.** Shift Your Thinking and Spending • 166
**126.** Define Your Role • 167–168
**127.** Keep Your Sanity • 169
**128.** Stimulate Your Mind • 170
**129.** It's Not All about Cooking and Cleaning • 171–172
**130.** Maintain Your Sense of Self • 173–174
**131.** The Importance of Alone Time • 175
**132.** Consider Working from Home • 176
**133.** Finding a Work-from-Home Position • 177
**134.** Hold Your Head High • 178
**135.** A Noble Job • 179

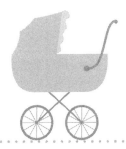

# Part 9

## Stay-at-Home Parenthood

Many modern mothers are choosing to stay home and not work when their children are young. In doing so, they fight stereotypes galore. The good news is that they also reap numerous benefits from their new adventures as stay-at-home parents. Despite the stereotypes, there are many rewards that come with this position. Not only do you get to watch your baby grow, but you also get to retain control of your little one's care during these first crucial years of development.

# 121. The Decision to Stay Home

The decision to stay home is an easy one when it is your choice. You may have decided long before you ever became pregnant that home was where you wanted to be when you had your own children. This does not make you old-fashioned, conservative, or any of the other labels that might be thrust upon you. You're simply a woman who knows what she wants.

The problem may come when you realize that your dream job isn't what you expected. Being a fabulous mother of three is an easy concept but a difficult task. Be cautious about forming expectations for being a stay-at-home mom. Talk to other mothers and take in both the good and bad observations. Ask them how their lives differ from what they expected. You'll hear some women complain about lack of sleep and others excitedly babble about their little one's latest accomplishment.

## If It's Not Your Choice 122

If you are required to stay home with your baby and it's not really your choice, you will certainly have a tougher time getting used to your new role. Sometimes this happens due to illness, location changes, job markets, or finances. Any of these situations can quickly find one or the other parent at home with the children, and many times this is the mom.

Your first instinct may be to grit your teeth and tough it out. This is a fine coping mechanism; however, it won't help for long. You need to either commit to being a stay-at-home parent or find an alternative solution.

## 123. Should Dad Stay Home?

Perhaps what works best for your family is for one parent to stay home. While many people assume this will always be the mother, your partner may be the better choice for a stay-at-home parent, depending on your situation. In choosing one parent over the other, there are many factors to take into consideration, such as the following:

- Who has more earning potential?
- Who has more job-growth opportunity?
- Who has the better/less costly insurance?
- Who is better suited to staying home?

If you have a very lucrative career in a quickly growing field, you may be very hesitant to leave your job. As long as you and your partner agree that his staying at home is the best option, this will work out just fine. And don't worry; even though your partner might not have your maternal instincts, he does have paternal ones. Any initial problems he has will soon disappear with practice.

## Take a Look at Your Finances 124

The money issue is often the deciding factor for most families when it comes to deciding if a parent should stay at home. Even if you desperately want to stay home, it may not be clear how your family can survive without your income. There may be a workable solution hidden beneath your doubt.

Though your family would lose your income if you stayed at home, the truth is that you would also be free of a few extra expenses. Sit down and think of all the things you'd no longer have to pay for if you didn't work, such as the following:

- Transportation: Whether your drive, carpool, or use public transportation, there are some fees involved. Gasoline, car maintenance, auto insurance, bus fares, or train tickets might be on your current list of expenses.
- Day care: Babysitters, nannies, or day-care services might eat up a huge chunk of your paycheck. As a stay-at-home parent, you would eliminate these expenses.
- Other hidden costs: Perhaps you eat out, get clothes dry cleaned, travel, or purchase supplies more frequently while working. While some of these expenses are tax deductible, you still spend a lot on random things.

## 125 Shift Your Thinking and Spending

You might find that no matter how much you wanted to stay home, it's a difficult adjustment for you and your partner. However, there are some things that you can do to make the shift more economically feasible. By lightening your load, you can make it more possible to enjoy your new job as a stay-at-home mom.

First, consider how you can reduce your spending. Can you consolidate your debt into one payment? Sometimes you can even get a better percentage rate when you do this. Can you refinance your home? Rates fluctuate, so sometimes you can get a better deal than when you first applied. This is a great way to put more money into your pocket every month.

Start planning menus to help you save on grocery bills. Some locations actually have online grocery shopping. While you may spend $5 on the service, you eliminate all impulse buying and you don't have to go inside the store. But even if that doesn't work out, planning ahead can keep you from spending more than you wanted and keep you from heading to a restaurant on a whim.

## Define Your Role 126

Your role as a stay-at-home mom is a different one than probably any other job you've had in your life. You don't really fit in with the working crowd. You're new to the mommy crowd. It is quite awkward at first. Once life settles down, you'll be fine. You just need to jump in with both feet first and hit the ground running.

### Wearing Different Hats

Going from having a defined title at your job to being a stay-at-home mom is a difficult transition. This is why defining your role is so important. Super-mom is not a title you want to even begin to try on, let alone earn. It is important that both you and your spouse are on the same page when it comes to sharing responsibilities.

One of the biggest subjects to discuss is what can reasonably be accomplished during the day. It is simply too much to believe that you can keep your baby well entertained and safe while maintaining a spotless household, paying the bills, grocery shopping, and cooking dinner every night. And don't forget the laundry!

Talking about your expectations is the only way to address the situation. If you don't discuss these issues, your life will quickly spin out of control. Your partner will expect one thing and get another. You'll be wondering why he's not helping, and he won't even know you expect help.

Play to likes and talents when divvying up chores. If he's a great chef, let him cook a couple of nights a week, while you supply the groceries for the meal and clean up. Or if you absolutely hate garbage and he absolutely hates laundry, trade! There are reasonable solutions that can be worked out when you put your heads together.

**Life as Full-Time Mommy**

While it may seem that all there is to being a stay-at-home mom are chores, this is far from the case. The tiredness you feel from all these responsibilities will instantly fade away when you look at your baby. After all, he is the reason you do all this work. In the end, you'll find it's absolutely worth it.

You may be itching to clean out a closet, but your baby is particularly needy that day. Maybe your baby is being so much fun that you can't tear yourself away to do laundry or clean a bathroom. Don't sweat it. The chores can wait. Make sure you find the balance that works for you and your family.

## Keep Your Sanity 127

In your new life as a stay-at-home mom, you may sometimes look around and realize that the only people you've talked to that day are under the age of one. Soon cartoons will become your favorite shows and you'll find yourself humming silly kids' songs in the shower. When you notice your motherhood taking over your life, it's time to take a break.

### Getting Out

The easiest way to stay sane is to occasionally get out of the house. This can mean going out to the mall to walk around or going to a park or library to read in peace. What do these activities have in common? The company of other people, of course. You can't just talk to your baby all day. You need to have adult conversations as well. So get out there and talk to people.

You can also try some organized activities for moms and babies. This can be music classes or baby gym classes. Perhaps you can find a mother's walking group or a playgroup for babies. There are many activities that you can find to do with other moms and babies. Whatever you do, don't hesitate to get out of your house. Getting out will help you keep your sanity and expose you to potential new friends.

# 128. Stimulate Your Mind

You probably remember being pregnant and feeling like you were losing brain cells faster by the minute. The early daze of postpartum feels much the same. However, your hormones do eventually settle, causing this feeling to occur less frequently. Once you feel you've regained some control, consider doing things to stimulate your brain while you're at home.

Reading is always a good way to relax and entertain yourself. If you are able to simply pick up a book and go, good for you. If you need a bit more motivation, try a book club, either online or at a local library or bookstore. Puzzles and brain teasers can also be a lot of fun to do. These keep your brain nimble and quick. They are also easy to do in terms of time, location, and money. You might like word finds or the crossword puzzles in your daily paper as well. There are also puzzle books, magazines, and websites where you can find more puzzles than you ever imagined.

### The Scholarly Route

While you may not consider yourself a scholar, attending a class a couple of times a week might be just what you need to stay intellectually stimulated. This can be any sort of class that tickles your fancy, from a literature workshop to a studio art class.

# It's Not All about Cooking and Cleaning

Do not be put off by the thought of staying home just because you don't like doing dishes, laundry, and other housework. The main focus when you stay home should be on caring for your family. Housework is a potential extra, but you'd be doing some even if you worked outside the home. Caring for your baby can be a lot of fun and very rewarding.

### Add Structure to Your Day

Structure can be something to help you figure out how your days will go. You may love a routine, and you are welcome to use the same theories when you have kids, but obviously, flexibility is a must. Find out what you like to do with your baby and plan for these activities.

When you get up in the morning, have a plan for what you'll do. Obviously, breakfast is one of the first items on your agenda. Will you immediately shower and get dressed, or will you play a bit with your baby first? Finding a rhythm that works for you and for your baby can help you approach each day with purpose. Some babies do thrive on routines, though not stringent ones, particularly when it comes to feeding.

Fill your calendar with fun and laughter, and don't be afraid to go out and have adventures. Just remember to alternate periods of play with periods of rest.

You can overschedule even a small baby. And, of course, you need your rest as well.

### What to Do All Day

When faced with the prospect of spending each and every day at home with your baby, you might become overwhelmed. What will you do all day, anyway? This is totally up to you, so be creative. Do you like to exercise? Does your baby enjoy the stroller? Try taking a walk with your baby. The more you walk, the more exercise you get. Turn each walk into a lengthy discussion of what you see. Every time you point to the neighbor's dog, your baby is storing the information. One day you'll be rewarded when your baby shouts out, "Dog!"

Remember that your baby learns through playing. This means that all the playing that you can do with your baby is a great learning opportunity for her. Singing learning songs, like the ABCs, or counting out the number of objects you lay on a blanket or the number of kisses you give your baby—these are all learning situations for her. They also tend to be fun for you.

## Maintain Your Sense of Self  130

You might have worried that becoming a mother would completely change your identity, and in a way, it did. You can't become a mother without making huge changes in your life. This is particularly true if you used to work and are now a stay-at-home mom. However, the person you used to be is not gone forever—she has just evolved.

This evolution takes time. Your transition to motherhood doesn't end when your baby is born. While the pregnancy does confer the rite of motherhood upon you, the growth over that first year is what changes you. There are ways to influence these changes so that you don't lose yourself.

**Time for Yourself**

Finding time for yourself can be difficult as a new mother. By the time you try to add the demands of being a daughter, a wife, a friend into the mix, you may feel that there is nothing left for you.

To ensure that this doesn't happen to you, set aside time for self. This can be merely ten minutes every day. Those first few days of motherhood you may decide to use this time to shower. As your baby grows and becomes less dependent, you can move away more easily. This enables you to get away and take time for yourself.

### New Hobbies

One way to get out a bit more often is to take up a hobby. You might have a hobby you've done for a long time and wish to continue. Perhaps you'll pick up a long-lost hobby. Or as you evolve as a mom, you might find that a completely new hobby interests you. Any of these options is fine.

There are many hobbies that you might find interesting. Scrapbooking is a natural extension of becoming a new mother. It's the perfect time to begin to chronicle the journey of your life and your family's life. If you like singing, look for a local non-professional or semiprofessional singing group that performs a couple of times of year. A reading group that meets monthly might be another great idea for you as a new mother.

## The Importance of Alone Time 131

You may find it hard to believe that your baby is not connected to your hip permanently. It is perfectly acceptable to get out of your house without taking anyone with you. Realizing this is one of the hardest hurdles you may face, unless of course the hardest hurdle you face is actually leaving the house. There will be days when you may consider begging your partner to watch the baby while you go to the grocery store alone. Alone has a whole new meaning now that you're a mom. When you start believing that the grocery store is a hot hangout, it's time to get out alone more often.

It can be difficult to leave your baby in the care of someone else, even if it is just your partner. Regardless, you need to get away. Your baby needs to learn that sometimes Grandma or Daddy or Aunt Rosie will be in charge. And certainly your partner needs to learn to take care of your child without your help.

It is understood that no one takes care of your baby quite like you do. But sometimes leaving your partner and the child alone is beneficial, despite harmless mistakes. Remember, you should not feel guilty about needing to be away for a while. To care for your family, you need to be in tip-top emotional shape. A moody, neglected mom can't help anybody.

## 132 Consider Working from Home

You might decide that you want the challenge or the money that working from home can provide you. Working from home can give you the best of both worlds, but it can also have some bad points. There is a fine line of balance that has to be met to make a work-at-home arrangement not only pleasurable but profitable as well.

The problem with working from home is time. Most jobs from home will require you to find the time to do them. Skip the tendency to put it off until bedtime. This will only make you cranky and push your body out of whack.

If you are going to work from home, most experts agree that you need to set office hours for yourself. This can be very difficult to do when you're dealing with a newborn baby. It does get easier as your baby gets older. Naps and routines do become more predictable, making it easier to say, I'm going to have office hours during nap times. Office hours might be when you make calls, do paperwork, or even complete your actual job.

Having the support of your partner is crucial to making an at-home job work. Be sure to talk to him about all the possibilities before you accept a new assignment. Having his support will make finding the time and the effort easier, not to mention curtail fights over your job.

## Finding a Work-from-Home Position 133

While staying home with your baby, you may decide to look for work that you can do at home. Whether it is freelance work, in-home sales work, or another job, you first have to find an opportunity that suits you. Keep your eyes and ears open for any job that fits your situation.

You can find job listings in most newspapers on a daily basis. The same can be said for local and national magazines. Their classified sections can be filled with work-at-home offers. You can find jobs doing anything from stuffing envelopes to making jewelry. Be very careful about jobs that ask you for money up front. Check out the business in detail. Ask to speak to employees. And remember, things that seem too good to be true often are.

However, there are plenty of legitimate businesses that need help on a part-time basis. Many of these jobs can be done in your home. If you can't find a job you're looking for, take inventory of your skills. Is there a business you could run from home? A product or a service you could sell? Do you have a way to market your service or product?

## 134 Hold Your Head High

There are some who feel that staying home and raising children is not hard work. Or they feel that it is work not worthy of smart women. The truth is, staying home is some of the hardest work you'll ever do. No one has the right to diminish your commitment and devotion to your family.

Believe it or not, there are people out there who will make rude comments to you about your choice to stay home. They might say things like, "You're too smart to stay home," "What a waste of a good mind," or "You'll be so bored." These small-minded people aren't able to see that raising children is a very important task that is best left to those who are smart and competent. Parents are not only caregivers but playmates, teachers, homemakers, and role models. Some argue parenting is the most important job in the world.

You can be prepared with a snappy comeback for when you hear these remarks, or you can take the high road and ignore the comments from people who don't understand. No matter how you choose to respond to the negativity of others, always maintain your confidence in your choice.

## A Noble Job 135

Children really are the future, no matter how clichéd that sounds. When children are given good, healthy starts in life, they grow up to teach the same qualities to their families. This helps them to be good leaders in the future. Your investment in your child is not only a great experience for you but also a contribution to the future of society. Parenting is a noble job; don't let anyone convince you otherwise.

The time you spend in the playroom with your baby may very well be preparing your child for the boardroom. Think of all the great things you learn as a child. You learn about sharing, being friendly, bargaining, and other negotiations. These are the skills that will guide your little one through school, friendships, jobs, relationships, and, one day, his very own family.

Staying at home works very well for many families. It can be fun, exciting, and cost-effective. Remember that your children are only young once; being with them as they grow is an investment in their future. Chances are you'd only regret missing these important years of your child's life, but you'll never regret being there for every exciting milestone.

- **136.** Consider Practical Matters • 182
- **137.** Dealing with Societal Pressures • 183
- **138.** Think about Age Difference • 184
- **139.** An Only Child • 185
- **140.** A Full House • 186
- **141.** What Will Another Baby Cost? • 187
- **142.** Plan for Costs of Two • 188
- **143.** What to Do about Fertility Issues • 189
- **144.** Plan Your Pregnancy • 190
- **145.** Work Toward Preconceptional Health • 191–192
- **146.** Pregnancy While Caring for Another Child • 193–194
- **147.** When to Tell Your Child about the New Baby • 195
- **148.** Research Sibling Preparation Classes • 196
- **149.** Books and Videos Are Available, Too • 197
- **150.** Enjoy Your Journey! • 198

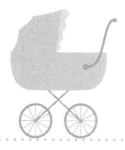

# Part 10

## Ready for More?

You've successfully survived the birth of your baby and the subsequent year. While it's been a year of changes, it has also been a year of growth. At some point during this time, you may begin to wonder if you'd like another child. This is a pretty common thought, even if it is not acted on. However, this is a big decision. There are certain questions you need to ask yourself and your partner before you even think about having another baby.

## 136 Consider Practical Matters

When trying to decide if you're ready for another baby, think not only of the high points of the first year, but the low points too. How did your first birth go? Are you ready to give birth again? Are you ready to lose sleep again? Do you have the physical and mental stamina to take care of two children, even if you will be working outside of the home?

What about monetary concerns? Do you have enough income to afford another baby? While you certainly can reuse many of the big-ticket items from your previous child, diapers are expensive!

There are also issues of medical care. Do you have insurance? What types of deductibles are in your policy? What will your out-of-pocket expenses be for this birth?

Once your new baby is here, how will you afford day care? Will it be less expensive for you to get a nanny? Perhaps the next child will be the one that breaks the budget and sees you considering staying home. There are many things to think about before having another baby. This is not to say that having another baby is a bad idea. It is just an idea that requires a lot of decisions.

## Dealing with Societal Pressures

Perhaps you feel like society is pressuring you to have more children. Maybe you've seen all the stories on late-night television about only children gone bad. Whatever your reason for wanting another child, you have to remember that it is yours and yours alone.

You need to not give in to societal pressures. Say no to your mother-in-law who really wants another grandbaby. Tell your child that Mommy and Daddy will be the ones to decide if they need another baby in the family. This can be hard to do.

The pressure we get from almost everyone is amazing. Once you have a baby, everyone automatically expects the next one to follow a couple of years later. And when that baby doesn't come, surely something must be physically wrong, because you obviously want another baby, right?

## 138 Think about Age Difference

Everyone will tell you that he knows what the perfect distance is between children. The truth is that there are benefits and disadvantages to nearly all age spreads. You need to figure out which of these benefits and disadvantages are most important to you, and which will have the most impact on your life.

The truth is that pregnancy can take a toll on your body. How heavy that toll is depends on multiple factors. If you had a relatively easy pregnancy, stayed healthy, and had a fairly straightforward and normal birth, you will have a much faster recovery than someone who was ill, in poor shape, or had a surgical birth.

If you gave birth by cesarean, it is imperative that you wait the requested eighteen months before becoming pregnant. Getting pregnant prior to this time gives your incision less healing time and may be associated with a greater risk of uterine rupture at the incision site.

Talk to your doctor or midwife to see if they have a recommendation about how long to wait between pregnancies. They may have medical reasons for you to wait longer or shorter periods of time. Your practitioner can base this on your personal medical history rather than reading a chart someplace. Being physically ready for a future pregnancy is very important, not only to your health, but to the health of the baby as well.

## An Only Child

You and your partner may decide that one child is enough for you. There are many families choosing to have only one child. Some benefits of having an only child are that more time, attention, and monetary resources are given to a single child since they are not divided among siblings.

Having an only child can be wonderful. You and your partner don't have to divide your time between other children and can focus on the one child. You can both go to the science fair or the school play and not tag team each other. Whatever your reasons for wanting an only child, remember that the decision is yours. Be careful to avoid pressure from family and friends who think they know what is best for you.

Perhaps the decision to have only one child was not your decision. It may have been made for you due to medical or other personal circumstances. This can be difficult to come to terms with, but families come in all shapes and sizes.

## 140 A Full House

Having a house full of kids can be a wild ride. The proponents of large families say that the sibling experience is not one to be missed. The interaction and love that goes on in large families is amazing. It's also quite the operational venture for the parents as well.

Larger families learn to cope with sharing parents among siblings. They also quickly learn to work together. Large families learn to share resources and take care of each other. If you came from a family that was larger, you may want either to have a larger family or to avoid one, depending on your particular experience within your family background.

But how many is too many? This is a very good question. The answer varies widely. The only ones who can decide how many children to have would be you and your partner. Ultimately, you shouldn't have more children than you can financially, emotionally, or physically manage.

While you may have an idea in your mind of the ideal family size, be flexible. Allow for a settling-in period after the birth of each child, and then readdress the issue of more children. This prevents you from finding yourself overloaded based on a random number you may have pulled out of your head long before your wedding night.

## What Will Another Baby Cost?

How much could a teeny, tiny baby cost? The answer is lots and lots of money! Many times you don't think of all the costs of having a baby when considering starting or expanding your family.

When you are considering having another baby and the discussion of cost comes up, be sure to address all of the needs of your new baby. Regarding just the pregnancy, you will need to consider the expense of prenatal medical care and figure in the cost of any additional maternity clothing. The good news is that you can save some money by recycling your old maternity clothes.

After pregnancy, the big costs of your new baby begin to add up. Child care may be the biggest cost of having another baby. You can save money by reusing some of the big-ticket items your older child has already outgrown. You may also be able to reuse some of the clothes, depending on the gender, size, and season of the births of your babies.

## 142 Plan for the Costs of Two

Having two children, even at different ages, can be a huge burden on the pocketbook. The good news is that with some planning, there are ways to make having two children affordable for most families. (And it doesn't even involve selling the first child!)

Child care may be the biggest expense when you have more than one child. Planning ahead and thinking about the placement of your children can help you. For many families with two children, it will be more cost-effective for one parent to stay home with the children.

If staying home is not an option for either of you, there are other possibilities. One great option is in-home care. This means finding a nanny or babysitter who can come to your home to watch your children. This can be a savings of time as well as money for you. Many families find that they spend less money by using an in-home care provider for their children.

# What to Do about Fertility Issues

If you had problems conceiving your first baby, you probably wonder if you will experience similar difficulties. The answer is maybe. It all depends on the diagnosis you have for infertility. Some conditions seem to go away miraculously once a pregnancy is achieved, while other conditions may have to be dealt with for every conception.

If you do require medical intervention to get pregnant, your reproductive endocrinologist or other specialist will be more than happy to help you achieve a second pregnancy. The more aggressive the therapy that you required the first time, the more likely you are to require therapy this time, though not always.

### Secondary Infertility

The rates of secondary infertility are hard to define because many women do not seek help for secondary infertility. After a year of failing to conceive in spite of well-timed intercourse and no birth control, you should seek help from your doctor or midwife. Depending on your age, they may begin testing right away or advise other, less invasive measures first.

## 144 Plan Your Pregnancy

The best things you can do if you are contemplating a second baby are to be healthy and to plan your pregnancy. Planning your pregnancy means that you are taking a proactive approach to becoming pregnant, not just becoming pregnant accidentally. While many unplanned pregnancies do turn out well, planning gives you the extra boost to keep you and your baby healthy.

The timing of your pregnancy may be important to you. You might be in a job where you have built-in time off, like a teacher or seasonal worker. Being able to maximize your built-in time off can enhance your use of your maternity leave. The hard part is that you can't always plan everything the way you want to plan it. You may be lucky enough to get pregnant right away or right on time, but a pregnancy could just as easily come before or after you hope.

The best way to help predict the exact time to get pregnant is to use some form of ovulation prediction. This can be done by taking basal body temperature or with store-bought individual ovulation prediction kits or other, more sophisticated kits to help you predict when you will ovulate. This certainly can't hurt your chances of becoming pregnant.

# Work Toward Preconceptional Health

Planning your health is a great way to prepare for your new baby. It also gives you something to focus on in the pre-trying phase. There are many ways to get healthy while planning your pregnancy.

A visit to your doctor or midwife will get you started on the right track. There, you can discuss lowering your risks of pregnancy complications prior to pregnancy. This is usually accomplished by being at an appropriate weight, eating well, exercising, and taking good care of yourself. You will also talk to your practitioner about the discontinuation of birth control in preparation for getting pregnant.

### Diet

Being at your ideal weight when you become pregnant can lower many risks in pregnancy. It can help you reduce the risks of some really terrible complications from pregnancy-induced hypertension to gestational diabetes. These complications can endanger not only your life, but also the life of your baby.

Your doctor or midwife can help you identify your ideal body weight and your body mass index (BMI). She will help you find additional help in planning your diet. This may include printed materials or books. It may also include a trip to the nutritionist.

The key to a healthy prepregnancy is eating a variety of fruits and vegetables in addition to protein and fiber. If you eat more whole foods and vegetables, you'll find that you not only lose any excess weight you may have had, but that you will also have more energy. This can be vital to you if you are going to be pregnant while dealing with another child, particularly if that child is a toddler.

**Exercise**

Exercise is vital to staying healthy. If you already have a workout regimen, then planning for pregnancy shouldn't be a huge issue. You will probably simply want to be sure that your workout is one that can be continued safely during pregnancy. To do this, simply share your routine with your doctor or midwife.

Perhaps you've never gotten into the swing of the exercise thing. This planning phase is the time to really get into it and start your routine. Your prepregnancy workout doesn't have to be wild or horrific. Be sure to include your family; this will help you keep up the routine.

Your workout doesn't necessarily need to be hard core. Start simply by walking around your block once a day. This will help get you moving. Getting moving is often the hardest part. From there, simply add on to your walk when you feel able to do so. For most people, this is when the old path is no longer physically challenging.

## Pregnancy While Caring for Another Child    146

Expecting a new baby is great! You are probably excited to be expanding your family. However, caring for a first child while pregnant with a second is very challenging. You probably thought you had the pregnancy thing down, but with your added responsibilities of caring for your first baby, things can get messy.

### A Different Ball Game

Pregnancy the second time around can be a whole new world. You may think you remember what it was like to be pregnant. However, having another child to care for can really throw a wrench into your plans.

Remember how, in your first pregnancy, you simply lay down to nap when you were tired? There will be none of that, unless you can convince your toddler to nap too. There are days when you will break every rule you ever set, like letting your toddler watch television for an extended period of time, just so you can catch a couple of winks on the couch.

You may find yourself comparing your pregnancies. If in your first pregnancy you felt movement at sixteen weeks, you may panic when week eighteen comes and goes without a flutter. You may also be more involved in your medical care during pregnancy, since you are now able to see the larger picture.

## 146

**Physical Changes**

The physical changes that one can usually expect during pregnancy aren't a huge shock the second time around. What might really shock you is how soon the changes seem to happen in comparison to your first pregnancy. You will probably find that you start to show much sooner with your second (or more) pregnancy. This is often thought to be because of the laxity of the uterine and abdominal muscles from the previous pregnancy.

The problem with the physical changes is getting around. You might think that's nothing new, but think of new duties that you have now with an older child. Do you lean over your car to buckle your child into a car seat? What about lifting groceries? Can you do that while holding your toddler's hand and minding your protruding belly? Try leaning over and giving a bath when you are nine months pregnant!

Fatigue will be one of the biggest issues you'll face. Your child doesn't understand why you aren't able to go to the park and run around every day like you used to do. Take a nap when you can. The same goes for sleeping in when you can. Don't hesitate to ask your partner to take over some of the middle-of-the-night or early-morning duties when appropriate.

# When to Tell Your Child about the New Baby

One of the most exciting parts of becoming a new mother all over again is making your child an older sibling. However, encouraging your child to welcome a new baby and preparing him to have a healthy relationship with his new sibling can be both fun and frightening.

There are many answers to the question of when to tell your child that there is a new baby on the way. Most families choose to wait until at least the end of the first trimester. While pregnancy loss is a normal part of life, it is terribly hard to explain to your children. (This doesn't mean that you shouldn't tell your child earlier if you want to.)

The biggest part of the decision of when to tell will revolve around your child. Part of that determination will be based on the age of your child. An older child can handle a deeper understanding of pregnancy. A younger child may be able to handle only a couple of months of notice prior to the birth.

Warning! Don't tell your child about your pregnancy until you're ready for the whole world to know about it. There is something about a secret this awesome that makes it impossible not to talk about. So if you don't want Grandma or teachers to know, don't tell your child.

## 148 Research Sibling Preparation Classes

There are many sibling preparation programs available. What you choose should be age appropriate. It should also match your values and ways of thinking when it comes to birth and parenting.

Sibling classes may be offered at your local hospital or birth center. You may also find a private educator who holds sibling classes. The majority of these classes are designed for children between the ages of three and seven. This does not mean that they would not have benefits for children of other ages.

Most classes cover a variety of topics. They may discuss what new babies look and sound like. Most classes will cover the dos and don'ts of having a new baby in the house. You may even find that the class offers a tour of the hospital or birth center. This can help make the separation from mom, even if it's only for a short time, a bit easier.

You may need to take special classes if you plan to have your child attend the birth of her sibling. There is no one right age for an older sibling to attend a birth; it depends more on the child. The big keys to a sibling's attending the birth are preparation for the birth, a support person solely dedicated to her, and that the child has the ability to come and go as she pleases.

## Books and Videos Are Available, Too

There are many books and videos that you can use to show your child some of the aspects of a growing family. Books are very widely available in many topics. You may decide to offer a variety of books to your child to see what appeals to him.

Pregnancy books are a great start to answer the inevitable series of questions that will follow your pregnancy announcement. There are some great books that describe how babies grow inside you. Kids of all ages are thrilled with these books. They also can help pass the long months ahead as you discuss what your baby is doing on a weekly basis. *A Child Is Born* by Lennart Nilsson is a parental favorite.

Books on new babies are also important. What is a day in the life of a new baby really like? Find books that talk about how your child may feel once the new baby gets here. Kevin Henkes has a wonderful book called *Julius, Baby of the World.* There are many books available on the subject of new babies.

There are also videos available. They range from the "favorite cartoon character gets a new sister" type to those featuring a variety of personified animals having babies. Kids are okay with this type of show, but they know that there is a huge difference between cartoons and real life.

## 150 — Enjoy Your Journey!

Deciding to have another baby can be a lengthy process. Are you ready mentally and emotionally? Is your body ready to have another baby? Or do you need to take some time to prepare your body? Once you do get pregnant, there's no going back. So be sure you're ready! Expanding your family is a lot of work, but it's also great fun. Do what you can to ensure every pregnancy is better than the last and that each child becomes comfortable in his role as a sibling. Above all, enjoy your journey!

# Index

## A

Abdominal muscles, 112
Acne, 103-4
Another baby, 198
   and age difference, 184
   considering, 183
   costs of, 187, 188
   planning for, 190
   and societal pressures, 183
APGAR scoring, 35
Au pair, 155

## B

Baby development
   assistance, 99
   month one, 81
   months eight and nine, 88-89
   months four and five, 84-85
   months six and seven, 86-87
   months ten through twelve, 90
   months two and three, 82-83
   problems, 98
Baby, what to expect from, 27
Babysitters, 157
Bassinets, 17
Baths, 46
Birth, 2-6, 25-41
   control, 134-39
   plan, 4
   preparing for, 26
Body
   after birth, 30, 102
   image, 120
Bone movement, 107
Books and videos, 197
Bottle choice, 72
Bottle-feeding, 71
   multiples, 73
Bouncers, 20-21
Breastfeeding, 44, 66, 108
   as birth control, 139
   multiples, 67
Breast
   leaks, 70
   pump, 68
Breathing difficulties, 38
Bringing baby home, 41
Budget, 10-11

## C

Cesarean birth, 32

Calories, 108
Caring for yourself, 117
Car seats, 15-16
   convertible, 16
   infant, 15
   toddler, 16
Child care, 150-51, 152-53, 154, 155, 156, 157
   costs, 158-59
Classes, 5
Condoms, 134
Co-sleepers, 17
Co-sleeping, 53
Cradles, 17
Creativity, 95
Crib, 17
   sleeping, 54
Cruising, 97
Crying, 51

## D

Day care, 152-53. *See also* Child care
Diapers, 47-48
   cloth, 47
   disposable, 48
   services for, 48
Doulas, 3
Dry skin, 104
Due date, 7

## E

Eating after birth, 62
Emotions, postpartum, 34

Exercise, 108, 109, 110-11
   clothes, 115
   at home, 113
   obstacles to, 114
   shoes, 115
Eye and ear screenings, 37

## F

Family
   child care, 154. *See also* Child care
   and Medical Leave Act, 8-9
Fathers, 149, 164
Feedings, 65
Fertility problems, 189
Flexibility, 112-13
Formula, 45
Front packs, 22

## G

Gyms and spas, 113

## H

Hair changes after birth, 105
Help after the birth, 12-13
Hips, 107
Hobbies, 174
Holding your baby, 50
Hormone fluctuations postpartum, 125
Hospital, tips for, 29

## I

Intrauterine device (IUD), 135

## J

Jaundice, 40
Job. See Work
Job sharing, 144
Johnny jump-ups, 21
Jumpers, stationary, 21

## L

Large families, 186
Losing weight after baby, 108

## M

Makeover, 120
Maternity leave, 8-9
Meal planning after birth, 64
Meconium staining, 39
Music, 59

## N

Nannies, 156. See also Child care
Newborn development, 80
Nutrition plan, postpartum, 63

## O

Only child, 185
Oral contraceptives, 135
Organization, 23
Outings with baby, 55

## P

Packing for the hospital, 6
Pain, 31-32, 33
Patch or ring contraception, 136
Pediatrician, choosing, 14
Periods after birth, 106
Pill contraception, 135
Plastic surgery, 116
Potty training for infant, 49
Practitioners for birth, 2-3
Preconception health, 191-92
Pregnancy
  while caring for another child, 193-94
  expenses, 10-11
Pretend play, 94
Pumping
  tips, 69
  at work, 143

## R

Reading to baby, 58
Ribs, 107
Routine, 56

## S

Savings, 11
Secondary infertility, 189
Separation anxiety, 146, 147
Sex
  desire for, 132
  first time after baby, 126

Sex—*continued*
   frequency, 133
   positions, 127-28
   readiness for, 121-22, 124
   and romance, 129, 131
   time for, 130
Sibling classes, 196
Six-week postpartum checkup, 123
Skin changes, 103-4
Sleep,
   crib, 54
   newborn basics, 52
Slings, 22
Solids, 76
Staying home, 148
   adjusting to, 167-68
   benefits of, 179
   decision to, 162
   and fathers, 164
   finances, 165
   not by choice, 163
   self image, 178
   spending, 166
   staying sane, 169
   stimulating your mind, 170
   structure, 171-72
Stocking up on essentials, 13
Stretch marks, 103
Strollers, 18-19
   carriage, 18-19
   double, 19
   jogging, 19
   umbrella, 18
Swings, 20

# T

Table food, 77
Tactile stimulation, 92
Talking to baby, 57
Telling your child about a new baby, 195
Time for yourself, 173-74, 175
Toys, 93
Tubal ligation, 138
Tummy time, 96

# V

Vaginal birth, 31
Vasectomy, 137
Visitors at hospital, 28

# W

Weaning, 74-75
   from bottle, 74
   from breast, 75
Weighing, measuring, and blood work, 36
Work
   alternative schedule, 144
   and balance, 145
   at home, 176, 177
   going back to, 142
   when to leave, 7. *See also* Maternity leave